Social skills and mental health

Social skills and mental health

Peter Trower, Bridget Bryant *and*
Michael Argyle, *with help from*
John Marzillier

University of Pittsburgh Press

Published in Great Britain 1978 by
Methuen & Company Limited
Published in the U.S.A. 1978 by the
University of Pittsburgh Press, Pittsburgh,
Pa. 15260
© *1978 Peter Trower, Bridget Bryant,*
Michael Argyle and John Marzillier

Library of Congress Cataloging in Publication Data

Trower, Peter
  Social skills and mental health.

  Includes bibliographies.
  1. Interpersonal relations. 2. Social interaction.
3. Mental health. I. Bryant, Bridget, joint author.
II. Argyle, Michael, joint author. III. Title.
HM132.T76   1978   158'.2   77–10544
ISBN 0–8229–1131–0

Printed in Great Britain by
T. & A. Constable Ltd, Edinburgh

Contents

Frontispiece

The Honourablest Part of Talke is to give the Occasion; And againe to Moderate and passe to somewhat else; For then a Man leads the Daunce. It is good, in Discourse and Speech of Conversation, to vary and entermingle Speech of the present Occasion with Arguments; Tales with Reasons; Asking of Questions with telling of Opinions; and Jest with Earnest: For it is a dull Thing to Tire. . . . He that questioneth much shall learne much and content much; But especially if he apply his Questions to the Skill of the Persons whom he asketh; For he shall give them occasion to please themselves in Speaking, and himselfe shall continually gather Knowledge. But let his Questions not be troublesome; For that is fit for a Poser. And let him be sure to leave other Men their Turnes to speak. Nay, if there be any that would raigne and take up all the time, let him finde meanes to take them off and to bring Others on. . . . And to speak agreeably to him, with whom we deale, is more then to speake in good Words or in good Order.

Francis Bacon: 'Of Discourse' 1597

Acknowledgements

The research on social skills training carried out at Littlemore Hospital, Oxford from 1968 to 1976 could not have been achieved without the help of many people. We are grateful to the Oxford Regional Hospital Board and its successor, the Oxfordshire Regional Health Authority, for their generous and sustained financial support, without which none of the work could have been done.

We should like to express our warm appreciation to our many colleagues and friends who gave their talents in various ways and at different times to the research. We are especially indebted to Krysia Yardley who was a member of the research team from 1972 to 1975 and whose combined interests in psychology and drama made a unique contribution to the development of the training; and to Felix Letemendia who helped to launch the research by taking clinical responsibility and entrusting us with some of his patients, and who continued to supervise, advise and support us throughout the period, as well as undertaking the clinical assessments. We wish also to thank Barbara Lalljee, Ruth Fearnley, Doreen Baxter, Florissa Alkema, Susan Martin and Phyllis Shaw who worked with us at various stages; and Elizabeth Chavasse, our secretary, who patiently typed her way through several drafts of the manuscript and generally organised our activities.

We are grateful to Andrew Mathews, who read the manuscript and, while not necessarily agreeing with us, helped us through his incisive and constructive criticisms to clarify and order our ideas.

Finally, we should like to thank those courageous individuals who agreed to undergo the training. It is not easy for those who are depressed or anxious to take part in research, but they not only accepted readily the arduous assessment procedures, but also contributed greatly to the development of the training through their own comments and criticisms. We wish them well, and sincerely hope that from our mutual efforts they may have reaped at least a few social rewards.

Part One

1 The social skills training approach

The definition and treatment of mental disorder has undergone considerable change in the last twenty years, due partly to new theories and discoveries in medicine and the social sciences. One trend has been towards training in new patterns of interpersonal behaviour. In this book we explore the progress that has been made so far with one approach in this field.

This is based on the idea that some forms of mental disorder are caused or exacerbated by lack of social competence, and can be cured or alleviated by means of training in social skills. There are two possible sequences of events. (1) Failure of social competence is primary, leading to rejection and social isolation, which in turn produces disturbed mental states. (2) Other kinds of mental disturbance affect all areas of behaviour, including social performance; social inadequacy results in rejection and isolation, thus adding to the original sources of stress and leading to deterioration.

The two main implications of this theory are that (1) certain groups of mental patients will be socially inadequate, and (2) they should improve or recover as the result of training in social skills. As yet there is no direct evidence on the aetiological sequences described above.

In this book we shall be looking at the evidence on these two

points, and will try to answer some of the following questions:
First, what is meant by social inadequacy? Chapter 2 describes
what is known about normal social behaviour and how this can
break down. Second, what are the causes of social inadequacy?
Chapter 3 reviews the work on the processes of successful and
unsuccessful acquisition of social skills in childhood and adolescence. Third, what are the characteristics of socially inadequate
people? Chapter 3 also looks at surveys of the way that socially
unskilled psychiatric patients actually behave. Fourth, what
techniques exist for improving social skills? The fourth chapter
examines therapeutic and other techniques, both new and old,
which are designed to alter and improve interpersonal skills.
Fifth, do these various therapies actually work? Chapter 5
examines the evidence from experimental studies on training.
Sixth, how is training actually carried out? The second half of the
book offers a practical assessment and training guide to therapists.

To help provide a framework for the book, the issues that each
of these questions raise will be briefly discussed in the rest of the
introduction.

What is meant by social inadequacy? A person can be regarded
as socially inadequate if he is unable to affect the behaviour and
feelings of others in the way that he intends and society accepts.
Such a person will appear annoying, unforthcoming, uninteresting, cold, destructive, bad-tempered, isolated or inept, and will be
generally unrewarding to others. It will be shown in chapter 2 that
these impressions (and their opposites) are conveyed to others by
the way in which 'elements' of behaviour are used – including
speech and non-verbal signals, such as looking, smiling, gestures
and so on. The socially inadequate person will be bad at using
these skills and at understanding other people's use of them. Many
people who are not psychiatric patients may also be rather bad at
this, and what distinguishes them from patients may be more the
degree of deficit than any qualitative difference – i.e. the extent to
which their inadequacy disrupts social life. The particular skills
which inadequate patients lack will be discussed in chapter 3.

Whether behaviour appears normal and acceptable to others
will depend on the customs and values of society, and some of the
implications of this for both assessment and treatment are also
discussed in chapter 3.

What are the causes of social inadequacy? Studies of social

learning suggest that social skills are acquired from childhood onwards, partly through *imitation* of others, including parents, siblings and peers; partly through *reinforcement* – i.e. encouragement or discouragement on the part of parents and others; partly through opportunity to *observe* and *practice* behaviour in a range of situations; partly through the development of *cognitive abilities*, and partly through *innate potential*. Social inadequacy may come about in a number of different ways. The relative importance of these influences and the exact processes involved are not fully understood, but some of the evidence is discussed in chapter 3.

Which kinds of patients are socially inadequate? Many patients are recognisable first and foremost through abnormalities of social behaviour. This may be failure to communicate with others, and some of the main symptoms are in the field of interaction and interpersonal relationships. Failure in non-verbal communication, for example peculiarities of looking, posture, gesture, facial expression, tone of voice and so on, together with incoherent speech, lack of affect, poor perceptual sensitivity and perhaps also poor empathic ability, have been found in schizophrenia and some kinds of personality disorders. Chronic schizophrenic patients probably show the most extreme forms of social inadequacy. Depressed patients also show poor verbal behaviour of a generally flat, passive and expressionless kind, lack initiative in conversation, adopt a helpless attitude towards the environment, and may lose interest in friends and social life. Anxious patients may show their anxiety in rapid and breathy speech which is interrupted by speech disturbances, and in tense posture and jerky and poorly controlled gestures, and they are often over-sensitive to the reactions of others, fear that they are saying or doing the wrong thing and dread being the centre of attention. Some develop phobias to specific social situations. Many psychiatric patients have distorted perceptions of their environment, paranoid interpretations being an obvious example; many are 'egocentric' in the sense that they lack the empathic ability to perceive themselves and the world from another's viewpoint. Some patients also have disturbed goals in their encounters with other people, for example aggressive and destructive ones.

Some forms of social inadequacy are not easily classified into diagnostic categories. In a survey of psychiatric out-patients we used the concept 'social inadequacy' as a category in its own right, and found a sizeable proportion – nearly 28 per cent of non-psychotic patients – could be reliably classified in this way.

How does social skills training compare with other approaches to this problem? Some dynamically oriented therapists believe that social inadequacy in patients is usually 'motivated', i.e. attains some goal for the patient, or is a result of inner conflict, and improvement can only come by resolving these underlying problems. We believe that disturbed motives and conflicts often result from frustrations in interpersonal relations, and that the best approach is to improve communication skills. It follows from the psychoanalytic position that social skills training would simply lead to the emergence of new symptoms, and not improve mental health at all. As we shall see in chapter 5, there is reasonable evidence that social skills training does improve mental health.

Social inadequacy is recognised within the behaviour therapy tradition. Here the emphasis has been on two main forms of failing, lack of assertiveness and social phobias. However, surveys of patients, reviewed in chapter 3, and our own experience of those who come forward for social skills training, show that mental patients display a much wider variety of forms of social inadequacy. These will be listed in chapter 2 and related to the different processes involved in the production of social behaviour. For instance, we shall show how failure in skills can occur at the cognitive and perceptual as well as behavioural levels, and how inadequate behaviour can be seen as a breakdown in the signalling system.

Social skills training is based on the idea that skills are learned and therefore can be taught to those that lack them. Effective social skills training has been made possible by recent advances in many fields of research. Considerable strides have been made by social psychologists, linguists and sociologists in the study of non-verbal communication, speech and conversation, the analysis of situations and other aspects of social behaviour. These are reviewed in chapter 2.

Studies by social and behavioural psychologists on the principles of skill acquisition, such as demonstration, practice and feedback, have provided insight into how behaviour may be learned, and are discussed in chapter 4. Applied studies in the field of psychiatry, education and management have attempted to put into practice and sometimes to evaluate the effectiveness of techniques for changing social behaviour, and these are discussed in chapter 4. Studies in developmental, social and abnormal psychology have provided clues about the origins of social development and possible reasons for the failure to acquire social skills, some of which are discussed in chapter 3.

Our own assessment and training procedures are a synthesis of many of these ideas and findings, together with the conclusions drawn from eight years experience with patients. These procedures appear as the second half of this book in a form which, we hope, will be of direct practical use to therapists in treating a limited range of problems in the field of neuroses and personality disorders. Our method can also be adapted for other patients, such as grossly deficient chronic schizophrenics who require a different form of training programme but with much the same content.

The form of social skills training that we recommend is different, in practice, from the procedures developed by some others, but the basic idea is usually the same. This is that patients or others deficient in skills can be taught directly a new and more socially accepted repertoire of skills, which will enable them to influence their environment sufficiently to attain basic personal goals. This *training* approach stands in contrast to other therapies, aimed at eradicating or inhibiting maladaptive behaviour or symptoms, or changing underlying neurotic defences and conflicts. Training does not preclude these other approaches, and our purpose is partly to explore fruitful combinations.

The concept of didactic training as a form of therapy has gained a good deal of ground in the last five years, and this trend has been reviewed by Authier *et al.* (1975) who state '. . . the educational model means psychological practitioners seeing their function not in terms of abnormality (or illness) → diagnosis → prescription → therapy → cure; but rather in terms of dissatisfaction (or ambition) → goal getting → skill teaching → satisfaction (or goal achievement)'.

Patterson and Carkhuff (1969) similarly state: 'Perhaps theory is not necessary! What we may need is direct training or education of everyone in the conditions of good human relations . . .'.

Finally, fellow social therapists Goldsmith and McFall (1975) write: '. . . in contrast to the therapies aimed primarily at the elimination of "maladaptive" behaviours, skills training emphasises the positive, educational aspects of treatment. . . . Whatever the

6   Social skills and mental health

origins of deficit (e.g. lack of experience, faulty learning, biological dysfunction) it often may be overcome or partially compensated through appropriate training in more skilful response alternatives.'

References

AUTHIER, J., GUSTAFSON, K., GUERNEY, B. AND KASDORF, J. A. (1975) The psychological practitioner as a teacher: A theoretical-historical and practical review. *The Counseling Psychologist*, 5, 31–49.

GOLDSMITH, J. B. AND MCFALL, R. M. (1975) Development and evaluation of an interpersonal skill-training program for psychiatric inpatients. *J. Abnormal Psychology*, 84, 51–8.

PATTERSON, C. (1969) Foreword to *Helping and Human Relations* (R. Carkhuff). New York: Holt, Rinehart & Winston.

2 The analysis of social behaviour

Introduction

Until comparatively recently, little was known about the elements and processes of social behaviour, and even less about how these might fail. Research and diagnosis were conceptualised in global terms, of personality, styles and traits, and abnormal forms of these. In the last two decades, however, there have been extensive new developments. Social psychologists have carried out experiments on gaze, facial expression and other aspects of non-verbal communication, 'taking the role' of the other, and the sequence of social events. Sociologists have pointed to the importance of self-presentation, the rules of social behaviour and the variation of behaviour from one situation to another. Linguists have examined the different functions of utterances as 'speech acts', the ways in which utterances form a conversation and the generative rules governing sentence construction. Anthropologists have shown how some aspects of social behaviour vary greatly between different cultures and subcultures, while other aspects are culturally universal. Philosophers have argued that the old, deterministic model of social behaviour was mistaken, and that people are to a large extent producing social acts which are intentional and consciously planned.

8   Social skills and mental health

Conceptual models are needed to integrate and make sense of these many findings. This book is concerned with one such idea – the social skills model – though other theories are also discussed. In this chapter we shall describe this model and list the kinds of failure which the model implies. We shall then describe the elements of social behaviour and show how they are organised into higher-order skills. Other implications of the model are developed, such as the role of gaze in synchrony and feedback, and social reinforcement.

The social skills model

This model conceptualises man as pursuing social and other goals, acting according to rules and monitoring his performance in the light of continuous feedback from the environment. This has some of the features of a serial motor skill (see chapter 4) and this analogy was put forward by Argyle and Kendon (1967). The model can be represented as in figure 2.1.

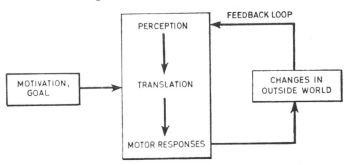

Fig. 2.1   Motor skill model

MOTIVATION, GOALS AND PLANS

The motor skill operator has definite goals – for instance to build something or to drive somewhere. People have social goals too: to make friends, to persuade, to extract or give information, to supervise others. These goals are desired because they provide outlets for basic needs – affiliation, achievement and so on. There are other similarities; the motorist has a final goal, for instance to drive to Aberdeen, and a number of subgoals, corresponding to places *en route*, or at an even smaller level, single adjustments of the steering wheel. Social goals are also hierarchically organised in this way. The longer sequences of behaviour are controlled by plans: a motorist plans the route to Aberdeen, a psychotherapist plans the stages of therapy. Such planning is conscious and may be conducted in words, but the shorter sequences are habitual and mainly unconscious. At the top of the hierarchy there are the conscious plans and at the bottom are the habitual responses.

Often, particularly in chronic schizophrenia, patients appear to have no social goals, and their behaviour is sometimes regarded as irrational or meaningless. (However, social withdrawal may protect these patients from further psychotic episodes and may be seen as a goal in this sense.) In less withdrawn patients goals are assumed to be latent but may be blocked. Failure in goal-seeking activity may occur for several reasons: (a) goals may be contradictory when needs conflict. Approach and avoidance activity is the paradigm case, where social interaction is desired but feared; (b) goals may be suppressed or extinguished because of a history of failure or a disturbance of mood, as in some forms of depression or schizophrenia; (c) when goals are blocked they may be converted into a different form, which may be both a poor and incapacitating substitute for the patient, such as obsessionality or sexual or other deviancy, or destructive behaviour towards others, such as the neurotic goals described by Berne (1966); (d) the cognitive skills required for planning may be inadequate. In recent experiments we have found that less competent students have shorter and less elaborate plans than the more competent. We have also observed that unskilled adolescent patients fail to develop the cognitive ability for generating plans and this seems to be related to a belief that they have no control over their environment (see pp. 30, 41).

PERCEPTION

The skilled manual operator must have accurate information on the task in hand, in order to decide what to do. This perception is highly selective and depends upon the plan he has in mind. This is also true of the social perceiver, except that his perceptual field is more complex and ambiguous, and the chance of mistakes therefore greater. What he attends to will depend, not only on his plans and motives, but on how well he knows the other person and situation, his social stereotypes, and his beliefs about the motives and plans of others.

Research has shown that there is great scope for misperceiving, particularly in unfamiliar settings, and mistaking cues in this way can lead to rapid breakdown in communication. Patients are often poor perceivers of other people, particularly of their feelings, schizophrenics again being an extreme case (Davitz 1964). There are several forms of failure: (a) low level of discrimination and accuracy; (b) systematic errors, e.g. perceiving others as more hostile than they are; (c) inaccurate stereotypes, or over-use of them; (d) errors of attribution, e.g. attributing too much to person, too little to situation; (e) halo effects, e.g. perceiving people as consistently good or bad.

TRANSLATION

Perceptions are 'translated' into performances, and the translation stage is a purely cognitive process which involves solving problems and making decisions. It involves a central store of information about possible causes of action; alternatives are considered and the best is selected in the light of previous experience. For instance, if a person talks too little, possible solutions are to use open-ended questions or give strong reinforcement, or if he talks too much, to use closed questions or no questions, negative reinforcement or interruptions.

Problems in this area are: (a) failure to consider alternatives; (b) failure to discriminate appropriate and effective actions from ineffective ones; (c) making decisions too slowly or not at all, perhaps due to uncertainty, or learned helplessness; (d) failure to acquire the right knowledge for making decisions, for instance, rules of conduct in social situations; (e) tendency to make negative decisions, due to poor self-esteem and negative self-instructions such as 'I can't do this.'

MOTOR RESPONSES

A repertoire of skilled behavioural responses is required, so that translation stage decisions can be implemented. As in the case of motor skills, these social responses are hierarchically organised, so that large units, like being interviewed, are composed of smaller units, like answering questions and single smiles and head nods. In learning a new social skill, it is often necessary to break a large unit down into its components, and learn each component separately. We shall discuss this aspect of training in chapter 4.

Patients show deficits at both levels, that is, of discrete elements such as gaze, facial expression, voice and verbal devices, as well as at higher order levels, such as warmth, assertiveness, and sequences such as social routines and basic conversation. These aspects will later be described at some length (pp. 49–53).

FEEDBACK

This aspect of perception occurs during the ongoing activity and completes the cycle. Feedback is received on the effect of actions and corrective action taken if necessary. This process of continuous monitoring allows for variation in the situation and errors in the initial plan of action. The kinds of failure that can occur include those listed under perception, and failure to attend to feedback. In addition there are problems in *giving* feedback: (a) there may be a lack of feedback, due to lack of skill or withholding of it for some reason; (b) it may be unrealistic or falsified, due, for instance, to neurotic needs and motives.

Failure at any point in the social skills cycle can lead to a worsening spiral of events, with inappropriate actions leading to more negative feedback, greater anxiety and withdrawal.

Elements of social behaviour

We said earlier that social behaviour is organised hierarchically, in that there are small behavioural elements, carried out more or less automatically and unconsciously, and larger units comprised of these elements, which are monitored according to a plan and ongoing feedback. We describe these elements in detail in our rating guide, page 156 ff., so deal only briefly with them here.

NON-VERBAL ELEMENTS

During social behaviour every part of the body is active. However, certain parts of the body convey more information than others, and do so in distinctive ways.

(a) Face. The face is a specialised communication area which is used by the non-human primates to express their emotional states and intentions towards other animals. In humans the face is more controlled but also communicates the main emotions and provides a rapid and continuous commentary on speech, for example by eyebrow raising and lowering. Information about personality and identity is also conveyed, for example by typical and idiosyncratic expressions and by grooming.

(b) Gestures. The hands communicate by illustration of the object of discussion, by pointing and by sign language. There is a close link between hand movements and speech. The hands also indicate the level of arousal, display truncated acts of touching, and 'autistic' gestures of self-touching, thought to show attitudes towards the self.

Other parts of the body function in different ways. Head nods, for example, indicate agreement, willingness for the other to continue speaking, and act as reinforcers. Bodily posture varies mainly along the tense–relaxed dimension: a relaxed posture is used by the higher status person in an encounter and comes to signal status. The feet do not convey much information, though they can indicate level of arousal, and individuals are found to have a characteristic set of foot movements.

(c) Gaze. The main function of gaze is the perception of non-verbal signals from others; in addition, the amount and type of gaze communicate interpersonal attitudes. Gaze is closely coordinated with speech, and serves to add emphasis, provide feedback and attention, and manage speaking turns. The different functions are combined, and a glance to collect information also sends information to the other person.

(d) Spatial behaviour. People communicate their liking for another by sitting or standing nearer and in a side-by-side orientation; status is signalled by distance and by using space symbolically, like taking the head of the table. Human beings establish territory like animals, though by different methods. They also control the behaviour of others by changing the spatial arrangements, for example by the position of a desk, and the style of decoration.

(e) Non-verbal aspects of speech. The same words can be delivered in quite different ways by variations in pitch, stress and timing. Linguists distinguish between 'prosodic' sounds, such as pauses, stress and timing, which affect the meaning of utterances, and 'paralinguistic' sounds, which convey emotions by tone of voice, and personality characteristics by voice quality, speech errors etc.

(f) Bodily contact. This is the earliest form of communication used by infants, and, probably for this reason, is a powerful signal in later life, indicating sexual, affiliative or aggressive attitudes. Bodily contact is controlled by elaborate social rules, and in western 'non-contact' cultures is only permitted in the family, at greetings and other ceremonies, by doctors and other professionals, and in anonymous crowd situations.

(g) Appearance. This is used primarily to send messages about the self. Styles of dress and hair, cosmetics and badges convey information about social status, occupation and personality, and constitute one of the main forms of self-presentation. Appearance also signals social attitudes, like sexual availability and rebelliousness, and emotional states. The meaning of these signals changes rapidly with time and fashion.

VERBAL ELEMENTS

The social functions of speech are now better understood, mainly as a result of work done by linguistic philosophers such as J. L. Austin (1962), who showed that many verbal utterances are 'speech *acts*' — they affect the behaviour of others as well as having meaning in themselves. Often the same message can be sent by a verbal or a non-verbal signal, for example saying 'yes' or nodding, saying 'over there' or pointing. There are several different kinds of utterance, which function in quite different ways:

(a) Instructions and directions are intended to influence the behaviour of others directly. Some of the earliest speech of children is of this kind, demanding food or toys. As well as specific instructions, there are 'structuring' utterances, as when a teacher indicates the nature of the next teaching episode. Instructions vary from commands or orders to mild suggestions.

(b) Questions are intended to influence verbal behaviour, i.e. to elicit appropriate replies. Questions are also used to initiate encounters: a reply indicates willingness to engage in an encounter. Questions also indicate interest in or concern for the other person.

(c) Comments, suggestions and factual information are given in response to questions, as independent comments on other utterances, and on special social occasions such as meetings and lectures.

(d) Informal chat or gossip. A great deal of social behaviour consists of idle chat, gossip and jokes, where little information is exchanged, and behaviour is unaffected. The purpose of these utterances is to establish, sustain and enjoy social relationships.

(e) Performative utterances. Many utterances have immediate social consequences, which constitute their meaning. Examples are naming babies, opening garden parties, giving verdicts, appointing to jobs, making promises, and apologising.

(f) Social routines. Greetings, farewells, thanks, and other social routines involve standardised verbal components, which have no meaning in isolation.

(g) Expressing emotional states, or attitudes to other people. Emotional states can be expressed in words ('I feel so happy'), but are more effectively expressed non-verbally, by facial expression and tone of voice. Similarly, attitudes to others present can be expressed in words ('I love you') but, as will be shown below, non-verbal signals have far more impact. Attitudes to people not present, however, are more commonly put into words.

(h) Latent messages. The same information, or questions, can be expressed in a large variety of different ways. One way may be chosen because it sends a further, implied message, for example about the importance of the speaker, or his attitude to the listener. ('Have you ever been to Nigeria?' 'No, that's one country I haven't been to.') Such latent messages may be intentional or unintentional.

Some psychiatric patients lack or over-use some of these verbal and non-verbal elements, and we shall review the evidence on this in chapter 3.

Organisation of the elements

Elements of behaviour are not usually used in isolation. Indeed, while some may have meaning in themselves (e.g. a wink, a clenched fist), most of them only have meaning in combination (e.g. the combination of raised brow, rising inflection, eye contact and verbal response in questioning) and when embedded in a sequence of responses (A makes a statement of fact or opinion, B questions this), and, at a higher level still, in a complete episode or several episodes over a period of time, such as in the stages of friendship. At the higher levels there is conscious monitoring according to a plan and the immediate feedback, and at lower levels whole chunks or units of behaviour are run off automatically. Faulty skills can occur at both these levels. At the lower levels elements may be combined in the wrong way or essential ones may be lacking, and because these habit patterns are usually over-learned and below the level of consciousness they are difficult to change. Our approach is to analyse these units with the aid of videotape, thus breaking them down into elements, bringing them to a conscious level and building them up again by training.

Even when these basic skill units are corrected, they may be combined wrongly at higher-order levels and be perceived as inappropriate in a given situation or stage in a relationship. Training at this level is concerned with effective plans and strategies to achieve desired goals, and involves the reorganization of behavioural units into a different sequence. In order to do this kind of analysis and retraining, we need to know how elements are combined in normal social interaction. The evidence on this will be reviewed in the next section.

ELEMENTS OF ATTITUDE AND EMOTION EXPRESSION

Attitude expression
Non-verbal elements are more important for interpersonal rela-tions, verbal ones for exchanging information and practical tasks. Argyle *et al.* (1972) found that if an unfriendly message is delivered in a friendly tone of voice and with a smiling face, the contents of the message are largely discounted, and the message is thought to be friendly. Similarly, verbal and non-verbal signals of superiority and inferiority were compared, and the non-verbal ones found to be much more powerful in affecting judgments (Argyle *et al.* 1970). These non-verbal signals also constitute a 'silent' or implicit language which largely – though by no means always – operates outside conscious control, in contrast to verbal language which is explicit and the focus of attention.

Another finding is that people can judge with some accuracy that others like them, but are less accurate in perceiving dislike. The reason for this is probably that expressions of dislike are largely concealed.

What are the major interpersonal attitudes and what elements of behaviour comprise them? Research has been conducted on both these questions. A number of studies have used ratings of different aspects of social performance and have commonly arrived at two dimensions (Foa 1961, Lorr and McNair 1965).

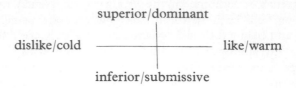

superior/dominant

dislike/cold ———————— like/warm

inferior/submissive

Our own and other studies have found inadequate and isolated people tend to fall into the dislike/inferior quadrant, unpopular leaders into the dislike/superior quadrant, good leaders into the superior/like quadrant, while popular, stable people are high on warmth and medium on superior/inferior.

Mehrabian (1972) looked at the elements which characterised these attitudes, and his findings are used in our manual. For instance, he found high or moderately high levels of the following elements were correlated with an affiliative style:

Total number of statements
Declarative statements
Questions
Duration of speech
Eye contact
Head nods
Pleasant facial expression
Verbal reinforcers
Positive verbal content
Hand and arm gestures
Pleasant vocal expression

Mehrabian also explored a cluster of non-verbal elements which he called 'immediacy cues', which, though they did not inter-correlate to form a single factor, together reflected a positive attitude, and were conceptually related in that they operate to increase physical proximity and mutual sensory stimulation. These cues may be conceptualised along a distant/intimate dimension, and include proximity, direct orientation, leaning towards, touching, eye contact.

Mehrabian and his co-workers found that cues of status (superior/inferior) did intercorrelate to form one factor, and were: asymmetrical limb positions, sideways lean and/or reclining position (seated), relaxed hands and neck. The related dimension of assertive/unassertive has been studied by Eisler et al. (1975), who found that high assertive subjects spoke at greater length and louder, with greater affect appropriate to the situation, smiled less, but had more speech disturbances.

Emotion

Emotions differ from attitudes in being subjective states of the individual rather than directed towards others, though emotions often become attitudes ('I am angry with you'). Like attitudes, emotions are mainly expressed non-verbally, but they are probably more conscious at certain stages of development and in certain situations, since there is a considerable amount of control of emotional expression. Another difference is that emotion is expressed mainly in the face and voice, while attitudes are expressed also by posture and position.

While the voice and face are the most important elements of explicit expression, other cues are important in modifying these, such as amount of gaze in intensifying (*more* gaze intensifies some emotions such as anger, *less* intensifies others, such as shame), and hands and feet are important 'cues to deception' (Ekman 1974).

Ekman and Friesen (1971) have put forward a model to help explain many of these facts. From their research on facial expression in five literate and two pre-literate cultures, they developed a 'neuro-cultural theory', in which 'neuro' refers to an innate 'facial affect programme' (the six primary expressions) and 'cultural' refers to events which elicit emotion and the cultural 'display rules', which are learned. This theory is shown in figure 2.2.

The theory has useful implications for the present approach. First, it implies that appropriate expression is a learned skill and can be assessed and treated as such. Second, it suggests specific ways in which expressions are managed appropriately or inappropriately. For instance, in some cultures men are expected to neutralise expressions of sadness and fear, winners or losers to deintensify expressions of happiness and sadness respectively. Third, the model can be applied usefully to other forms of emotion expression, such as the voice. Fourth, it directs us to ways of improving perception and expression of emotion by using specific and known display patterns. Finally, it draws attention to the role of other non-verbal elements in 'leaking' emotions which are facially controlled. An example of this occurs in anxiety, revealed by the hand activities which Ekman and Friesen call self-adaptors,

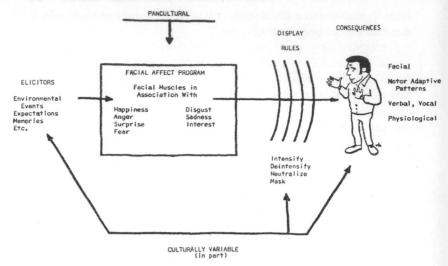

Fig. 2.2   Ekman and Friesen's neuro-cultural theory of facial
expression (after Ekman and Friesen 1971)

such as scratching or picking or covering part of the face.

Many of the non-verbal elements which comprise particular emotions are given in the manual and rating guide and need not be repeated here.

The expression of emotions and attitudes can go wrong in several ways:

1. Expression may be completely inhibited or unrestrained by over- or under-use of display rules. The former results in a neutral or blanked expression and flat tone of voice, so that no-one can tell whether a person is happy or sad, or whether he likes those present or not. This ambiguity can easily result in misinterpretation by others.

2. Expression may be predominantly negative or unpleasant – hostile, sarcastic, superior, and so on.

3. The wrong display rules may have been learned, resulting in expression of affect inappropriate to the situation. Linked to this is the problem of lack of awareness of expressions, or a mistaken belief about the expression being displayed. Points 2 and 3 often combine, in that there is a breakdown between the intended and actual expression, the intended expression being friendly, the actual one hostile or fearful. A common occurrence is for A to feel

friendly but anxious towards B, and to express only anxiety which is perceived negatively by B.

Expressiveness can be improved by increasing awareness of cues with video feedback and instruction, practice of the relevant facial muscles or the voice to correspond to the felt emotion, and learning appropriate display rules. Perception can be improved by exercises in interpretation, and by increasing awareness of the cues to concealed emotional expression.

ELEMENTS OF CONVERSATION

Just as elements are combined hierarchically to form higher-order units in attitude and emotion expression, so they are combined to form utterances, episodes and other larger phases in conversation. While non-verbal elements predominate in the former, verbal and non-verbal elements are equally involved in conversation, and they are organised quite differently and serve different functions.

Vocal and kinesic elements which affect the meaning of utterances
A person would not be accepted as speaking a language properly, indeed he would scarcely be understood, if he did not deliver his sentences in the vocal pitch-pattern, stress-pattern and temporal pattern of grouping and pausing proper for that language. The meaning of an utterance depends on the way it is spoken — particular words may be emphasised ('they are shooting *dogs*'), or formed into a question (usually by a rising pitch), and the whole utterance 'framed' by tone of voice, showing whether or not it is to be taken seriously, is meant as a joke, is sarcastic and really means the opposite, etc.

Similar considerations apply to kinesic signals (bodily movements), which can affect the meaning of a sentence by (1) providing the punctuation, displaying the grouping of phrases, and the grammatical structure, (2) pointing to people or objects, (3) providing emphasis, (4) giving illustrations of shapes or movements, (5) commenting on the utterance, e.g. indicating whether it is supposed to be funny or serious.

Graham and Argyle (1975) found that hand movements added to the efficiency with which two-dimensional designs and shapes could be communicated; they added more information for shapes which it was difficult to describe in words. These effects were greater in Italy, where hand movements are more pronounced, than in England.

Birdwhistell (1970) provided a system for recording kinesics on the analogy of the transcription methods used in phonetics; and Scheflen (1965) postulated that non-verbal communication has a hierarchical, three-level structure corresponding to sentences, paragraphs and longer sequences of speech.

It has been found that bodily movements are closely coordinated with speech in that a sentence may be accompanied by related hand or head positions. These movements also have a hierarchical structure, in which smaller verbal and bodily signals are organised into larger, and coordinated, groupings of both. Later research has shown that the coordination of bodily movements and speech is not as close as previously thought, though bodily movements do start at the beginning of spoken sentences and phrases. Since most of these movements can only be seen in peripheral vision, their function is rather mysterious. Kendon (1972) suggests that in addition to displaying the structure of utterances, these movements (1) make the speaker more interesting, and hold the listener's attention, and (2) give advance warning of the kind of utterance that is to come.

Elements which synchronise the interaction
In addition to his own performance – the expression of emotions and attitudes and uttering well-formed speech – the individual has to accommodate to the other by the feedback process referred to earlier in the description of the social skills model.

The social skills model suggests that the monitoring of another's reaction is an essential part of social performance. The other's verbal signals are mainly heard, but non-verbal signals are mainly seen, and this underlines the importance of gaze in social interaction.

One of the most important functions of gaze is to synchronise the behaviour of two or more people interacting. A study by Kendon (1967) showed that long glances are given by a speaker at the end of an utterance, and found that if a terminal gaze was not given by a speaker, there was a long pause before the other replied. It looks as if the terminal gaze is used as a synchronising signal, though it is primarily used to collect feedback on the listener's reactions.

Although people look in order to collect information in this way, the act of looking also sends information to the other. Argyle *et al.* (1973) separated the different functions of gaze in an experiment in which two persons conversed across a one-way screen. It was found that A (who could see) looked 65 per cent of the time, while B (who could not see) looked 23 per cent of the time, which suggested that A was looking to collect information; B's behaviour suggested that he was looking to send information. A looked more during ordinary conversation than during a mono-logue, when he looked only 47 per cent of the time; this difference was attributed to the need for more feedback and synchronising signals during a conversation.

When two or more people are conversing, they take it in turns to speak, and usually manage to achieve a fairly smooth 'synchronis-ing' sequence of utterances, without too many interruptions and silences. When people first meet, it is unlikely that their spon-taneous styles of speaking will fit together, and there is a period during which adjustments are made – one person has to speak less, another has to speak faster, and so on. This is all managed by a simple system of non-verbal signalling, the main cues being nods, grunts and shifts of gaze. For example, at a grammatical pause a speaker will look up, to see if the others are willing for him to carry on speaking – if they are, they will nod and grunt. Just before the end of an utterance a speaker gives a rather more prolonged gaze at the others. If this system fails interruptions will take place, and there is a struggle for the floor (Kendon 1967). Details of other signals used for synchronising are given in our Manual (p. 224 ff.).

Frame-by-frame analyses of small movements of hands, head, eyes, etc. in relation to speech, have also provided evidence of a different kind of 'interactional synchrony', i.e. coordination of bodily movements between speaker and listener over periods of time corresponding to sentences, and even to words (Kendon 1970, 1972).

The feedback system.   A speaker needs intermittent, but regular, feedback on how others are responding, so that he can modify his utterances accordingly. He needs to know whether the listeners understand, believe, disbelieve, are surprised or bored, agree or disagree, are pleased or annoyed. This information could be provided by *sotto voce* verbal muttering, but is in fact obtained by careful study of the other's face: the eyebrows signal surprise, puzzlement, etc., while the mouth indicates pleasure and displeasure.

The listener, for his part, must provide this intermittent evidence that he is still attending if the conversation is to be sustained. If a listener turns his back or falls asleep, the other will assume that he has withdrawn from the encounter. To signal attentiveness, listeners use (a) *proximity* – they are within the conventionally prescribed range, (b) *orientation* – they are appropriately oriented for the encounter in question, (c) *gaze* – they look at the speaker frequently, (d) *head nods* – used frequently, (e) *posture* – they adopt an alert, congruent or forward posture, (f) *bodily movements* – these reflect or mirror the verbal and non-verbal signals of the speaker.

When these signals are unavailable, as in telephone conversations, more verbal signals are used: 'I see', 'really', 'how interesting', etc.

The combination of verbal and non-verbal signals appears to go wrong in any patients who seem unable to maintain a conversation – which simply comes to a stop after the exchange of one or two utterances. The precise causes of failure are not known in detail, but the following seem likely:

1. Inappropriate use of verbal elements, not asking questions, not responding appropriately to previous moves by the other, or producing utterances that do not lead to obvious replies, such as uninformative statements.

2. Not using or responding to synchronising signals.

3. Failing to provide or respond to feedback and attention signals.

REWARDINGNESS AND CONTROL

People don't simply speak and mesh smoothly in conversation; they also reward and control each other. This brings in another aspect of the social skills model – motivation and planning – though the actual behaviour is executed often quite unconsciously at the 'translation' stage.

During social interaction, participants behave with differing degrees of rewardingness and control. This has two effects –

controlling the immediate behaviour of others, and affecting how much one is liked or disliked.

Many experiments have shown that if A follows some kind of behaviour of B's with smiles, head nods, gazes, or approving noises, B rapidly increases his production of the behaviour in question. If A frowns or gives other negative reactions, B reduces the amount of this behaviour. Almost any aspect of B's behaviour can be influenced in this way. The effect is markedly greater if B is aware which behaviour is approved or disapproved of, but a number of studies show that the effect can occur outside B's awareness. The effect is usually very rapid, and occurs in under a minute. People do not often produce systematic reinforcement deliberately, though they can do so, for instance, an ingratiator smiles and flatters preparatory to asking a favour. In ordinary conversation, participants are simply reacting positively or negatively to what pleases or displeases them in the other's behaviour. And the effect works in both directions: while A is influencing B, B is also influencing A. This is one of the main processes whereby people are able to modify each other's behaviour in the desired direction. Clearly, if people do not give clear, immediate and consistent reinforcements, positive and negative, they will not be able to influence others in this way, and social encounters will be correspondingly more frustrating and difficult for them. This appears to be a common problem with many psychiatric patients, who characteristically fail to control or try to over-control others.

The second aspect of rewardingness is its effect on the attitude of liking and disliking on the part of others. In a celebrated study of girls at a reformatory, Helen Jennings (1950) found that the popular girls helped and protected others, encouraged and cheered them, made them feel accepted and wanted, controlled their own moods so as not to inflict anxiety or depression on others, and were concerned with the needs and feelings of others. In other words, the popular girls were rewarding in a variety of ways. The unpopular girls did just the opposite – they were boastful, demanded attention and tried to get others to do things for them – they were trying to extract rewards, at a cost to others. There are a number of different sources of popularity and unpopularity but there is little doubt that being a source of rewards is one of the most important (Rubin 1973). One of the most common characteristics of socially unskilled patients is their low rewardingness; this is particularly the case with chronic schizophrenics, who have been described as 'socially bankrupt' (Longabaugh *et al.* 1966).

Putting together the two effects of rewardingness and control, it follows that to make friends *and* influence people it is necessary to give clear, immediate and consistent rewards when others act as desired, and to keep punishment for undesired behaviour to a minimum. Studies of leadership show that in order to be both an effective leader and to be popular, it is necessary to give directions in a special way – using the democratic/persuasive style: others are consulted and persuaded, rather than just being told what to do (Argyle 1972).

The actual behavioural elements have been listed separately in the manual as two main styles, and exercises are given for their use, both independently and in combination.

EMPATHY, AND TAKING THE ROLE OF THE OTHER

The social skills model gives a rather psychopathic view of social behaviour – suggesting that people are constantly trying to manipulate others as if they were cars or typewriters. It is a matter of common experience, however, that we are concerned about the feelings and thoughts of others. A cyclist is not constantly wondering how the bicycle is feeling, or whether it thinks he is riding it nicely. In conversation, however, we are concerned with what others are thinking, and to a greater or lesser degree imagine them to be socially skilled individuals with motives of their own. An individual may be worried about what sort of impression he is making (if being interviewed or assessed), what the other person really wants (if he is a salesman), or what the other's problems are (if he is a psychiatrist). He may do this in an external, calculating way, or he may find himself identifying with the other and sharing his emotions and problems (Turner 1956). A selection interviewer or social worker may start by doing the first, and end up by crossing over to the client's side, and trying to get him the job, or defending him against all comers. In many such encounters a balance has to be kept between sympathy and some degree of detached objectivity.

The ability to see another's point of view appears to be a cognitive ability which develops with age, but which may fail to develop properly. There are tests for the ability to 'take the role of the other'. In the 'as-if' test, subjects are asked to describe how their life would have been different if they had (1) been born a member of the opposite sex, and (2) been born a Russian (Sarbin and Jones 1956). It has been found that people who do well at such tests also perform better at laboratory interaction tasks. It is supposed that A will interact better with B if A can imagine correctly what B's point of view is – the problems he faces, the pressures he is under, etc. On the other hand, most people seem able to deal perfectly well with the opposite sex, and with older people – roles of which they have no experience, and which they probably imagine very inaccurately.

Failure to take the role of the other appears to be a common feature of psychiatric disorders. It is a familiar clinical observation, and Meldman (1967) found that psychiatric patients talked about themselves more than controls did. This could be a result of the clinical situation, since therapy often requires increased concern with the self. Our experience of socially unskilled patients, however, is that even outside therapy they find it difficult to see another person's point of view, and do not show interest in others.

SELF-PRESENTATION

The individual not only takes the role of the other, but imagines how the other perceives him as a person or 'self'. The average individual is perceived and treated in a fairly consistent way by other people; this is one of the main ways in which he acquires a stable self-image, and some measure of self-esteem. We are not concerned here with the structure or dynamics of the self-image, but rather with the characteristics of social behaviour in the area of self-presentation.

'Self-presentation' refers to the behaviour people use to communicate their self-image to others. This is a necessary aspect of social performance since it is very difficult to deal with another person unless enough information about him is made available – so that he can be treated appropriately. If an individual wants to be treated as a member of a certain occupation, social class or nationality, or as a particular kind of personality, it is up to him to send the relevant social signals. There are additional reasons for self-presentation in many professional jobs; it is often necessary to inspire confidence in others by looking, for example, like a bank manager rather than a revolutionary (or vice versa), by sounding like a teacher who knows what he is talking about, and so on.

Self-presentation is a social skill and requires special social signals. Much of it is non-verbal, the main signals being clothes, accent and manner of speaking, and general style of behaviour. The two strongest cues for social class in Britain, for example, are clothes and accent (Sissons 1970).

Jones and Gergen (Gergen 1971) found some of the rules of verbal self-presentation. They examined the speech of subjects who were motivated to convey a favourable impression of themselves. It was found that if they had higher status than the person addressed the subjects were modest, while if they were of lower status they drew attention to their assets but in unimportant areas. Subjects were modest if they believed that the other person was modest, and would admit their shortcomings if they anticipated a situation where compatibility was important. Verbal self-presentation has to be carried out with some subtlety, and usually very indirectly, or it becomes boastful and is greeted with derision and disbelief, in many cultures.

There are several ways in which self-presentation commonly goes wrong in 'normal' people.

(a) Audience anxiety. It is normal for inexperienced people to feel anxious when presenting the self in front of audiences. This usually, but not always, passes with experience, perhaps as a result of acquiring increased skill. This condition may require treatment if a person's job requires public performances and anxiety does not decrease with normal exposure.

(b) Embarrassment is a form of acute social anxiety which is precipitated by social events. Goffman (1956) suggested that it is due to the unmasking of bogus self-presentation, and later research has shown that this is one important source of embarrassment. Other causes are accidents which give an impression of clumsiness, such as falling over or dropping things and social *gaffes* like mistaking one person for another and forgetting someone's name.

(c) Deception and concealment. We have just seen that deception can lead to embarrassment. On the other hand, most people present themselves a little better than reality. Concealment of discreditable aspects of the self, as of negative attitudes towards others, is an essential part of life.

Self-presentation may go wrong in psychiatric patients in several ways.

(i) There can be a failure to emit enough information about the self; the individual appears 'grey', 'colourless', 'lacking in personality'.

(ii) He works too hard at self-presentation, over-dramatises himself, wants to be the centre of attention, and is constantly reminding others of his attributes.

(iii) He presents an image which is bogus, claiming to be more important than he really is.

(iv) He presents an image which is simply inappropriate, though not particularly prestigious. This may be due to a strong identification with some significant other person in the past or present.

Behaviour in specific situations

So far we have described the verbal and non-verbal elements and the psychological processes which they combine to form, and these are basic to all social behaviour. However, social behaviour takes place in specific social situations, and for each situation there are a restricted number of social acts, or moves, which are relevant and allowable.

THE RULES OF SITUATIONS

In every culture there are rules governing behaviour in most common situations. Unless all those present agree on the definition of the situation and the rules to be followed, chaos will ensue. Just as two people must agree to play the same game, e.g. tennis, rather than two different games, e.g. tennis and crocquet, so must they agree on the social situation they are in. As in the case of games, it seems that rules develop in the culture since they provide a satisfactory way of handling interaction in particular situations. In games there is a clear distinction between rules, such as the number of balls to an over in cricket, and conventions, for instance what kinds of trousers players should wear. The rules of the game give a meaning to many of the acts which take place, and the game can only be understood in terms of the goals and concepts involved in the game. Barker and Wright (1954) found that in a town in Kansas there were over 800 standard 'behaviour settings' – going to church, going to the drug store, etc., each of these situations having its own rules. We can discover which rules are essential by breaking them to see what happens.

In recent studies of social rule breaking we have found that the distinction between rules and conventions is an important one. Rules seem to be obligatory in each situation, the conventions not so. For example, at an interview it does not really matter if the candidate wears a sports jacket rather than a suit (convention), but it does matter if he asks all the questions or refuses to speak at all (rules). Similarly, a guest at a meal will be forgiven for using the wrong knife and fork, but not for refusing to eat or being rude to the other guests (Argyle 1975).

There are rules governing who may be present, the appropriate setting or equipment, the task and how it should be done, the approved topics and style of conversation, the interpersonal relationships and emotional tone, and sometimes the clothes worn.

There are also less obvious rules governing the sequence of individual utterances in different social situations, and it is useful to distinguish four kinds of combination (Jones and Gerard 1967).

1. Reactive contingency. Each person responds to the last move by the other. This applies to most impromptu social conversation, e.g. in pubs, coffee breaks and so on.

A R_1 R_3

B R_2 R_4

2. Asymmetrical contingency: A reacts to B, but B does not react to A – he is following a plan of his own.

A R_2 R_4

B R_1 R_3

This applies to some kinds of interviewing and teaching and to giving a speech.

3. Mutual contingency. Each person reacts to the other, but also has a plan.

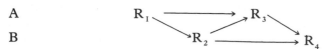

This applies to joint discussion, negotiation, teaching, therapy, and all situations where each person has plans of his own.

4. Pseudo-contingency. Each person is not really responding to the other, except in respect of timing, but is acting out a learned sequence. This applies to actors in a play, and to performers in a ritual, such as weddings and funerals and other highly structured interactions such as greetings.

At a higher level of organisation, strings of utterances, or 'moves', are formed into episodes bounded by a theme, such as a topic of conversation or having a meal. Each episode has rules governing behaviour within it and an internal sequence which is highly predictable, and participants cooperate to perform it as a joint social act. They will agree to enact a particular episode if this is expected to be sufficiently gratifying for each of them, though there is some scope for negotiating the way the episode goes. Social performers try to bring about certain episodes, which will produce the responses they are seeking. And there are rules governing the sequence of episodes. There are signals, both verbal and non-verbal, for introducing and negotiating the sequence of episodes. In asymmetrical contingency one person has a plan, in mutual contingency both have plans, which must be coordinated into a single joint plan.

At a higher level still, episodes form yet longer sequences or presentations, which may be a complete conversation, and which may extend over several encounters. Scheflen (1965) was the first to suggest this kind of hierarchy, though it is still a matter for investigation where the points of demarcation occur.

The above ideas have been useful in analysing the sequence of social behaviour in different situations, and seeing how failures can occur.

In the classroom, for example, the following moves have been distinguished. *Teacher*: responds sympathetically to expressed feelings, praises or encourages, accepts or uses ideas of pupils, asks questions, lectures, gives direction, criticises pupil or justifies own authority. *Pupils*: talk in response to teacher, or initiate talk (Flanders 1970). This list shows that the moves which can be made are different for teachers and pupils, i.e. for those performing different roles. Failure to follow them can result in silence or confusion.

There are several ways in which social competence may fail in the area of social rules.

1. Not knowing the range of social acts which are appropriate and meaningful in a situation. Candidates at interviews may engage in light-hearted chat, a guest at a party may engage in deep religious-philosophical interrogation.

2. Not being aware of the contingency structure of a situation. Socially inadequate patients appear to treat situations as if they are all of type 2, i.e. fail to pursue plans of their own.

3. Patients often report great difficulty with particular situations, or classes of situation. Often this appears to be due to a failure to understand some aspect of the rules, about what is expected, and what can be expected of others. Young people often find parties difficult, since they have not mastered the procedures for starting and stopping encounters with strangers.

4. Inability to use meta-signals to negotiate mutually agreeable episodes.

PERSONS AND SITUATIONS

We know from the work of Mischel (1968) and others that individuals are far from consistent between different situations. In the first place, situations are important determinants of behaviour – everyone is more anxious when sitting on a big dipper than while sitting in a deck chair. But in addition, different people are affected differently by different situations – some are made anxious by audiences, others by heights. In other words, behaviour is a function of persons, of situations and of person-situation interaction. Problems can arise if persons fail to behave differently in different situations, and Moos found a sample of mental patients to be *more* consistent than normals and to become less so as they recovered (Moos 1969).

Another approach to this problem is in terms of the internal – external control dimension. Inner-controllers feel that they can control events, and that what happens is mainly due to their efforts. External-controllers feel that what happens is outside their control and mainly due to chance or to other people. Some 'patients are found to be external-controllers (Lefcourt 1972).

Putting this finding together with the previous one, we can speculate that a causal circle exists between disbelief in the ability to influence events and failure to produce adaptive behaviour.

Undue emphasis has previously been placed on personality,

which has hampered both assessment and behaviour change programmes. For instance, personality questionnaires have been based on the belief that personality characteristics will account for most of a person's behaviour in most situations, and failure to predict behaviour has been put down to error in the measuring instrument. Similarly, newly learned behaviour in one situation usually does not transfer to other situations, and this is described as a 'failure to generalise'. It seems probable, however, that stable aspects of persons (P) interact with properties of situations (S) to generate particular behaviour in those situations, a proposition which may conveniently be designated as 'P × S interaction'. This view leads to a different kind of assessment and treatment approach and different expectations of outcome from previous ones, based on the variables, and may be attributed to persons and to situations. Some of these are listed below.

Each person variable is associated with a characteristic behaviour pattern, for instance, 'middle age' with a certain style of dress, behaviour and attitudes, 'working class' similarly with a style of dress, language and accent and other behaviour. Likewise, each situation variable prescribes and allows certain behaviours and appearances and disallows others.

Person variables (examples of)
(a) Demographic
   age
   sex
   culture and class
   marital state
(b) Physiological
   arousal level
(c) Personality
   extraversion
   neuroticism
(d) Motivational
   needs
   goals
(e) Cognitive
   attribution tendencies (e.g. internal v external control)
(f) Emotional
   anxious
   depressed

(g) Behavioural repertoire
   social skills
   behavioural styles
   (e.g. assertiveness, friendliness)

Situation variables

(a) Goals and task
   eating
   buying
   working

(b) Social themes
   social/cooperative
   male/female relations

(c) Rules
   e.g. for eating :
   time
   order of courses
   dress
   type of conversation
   seating

(d) Roles
   e.g. for eating :
   hosts
   guests
   senior/junior
   male/female

(e) Moves
   e.g. for eating :
   host greets and seats guests, serves food, initiates conversation

(f) Setting
   type of room, lighting, type of occasion (Argyle 1976)

Person × situation interaction

The person brings certain behavioural tendencies to the situation, while the situation, as we noted above, prescribes and allows certain patterns of behaviour. The way the two combine is complicated and in practical terms they are extremely difficult to separate. Research into the analysis of situations is still in its infancy and more research is needed before the P × S formula can be adapted for practical use in assessment and training. However, this and similar ideas have influenced clinical approaches and we have used some of them in our own assessment and training.

CULTURAL AND SUB-CULTURAL VARIATIONS

Social behaviour varies not only between situations but also between cultures and between social classes, racial groups and age groups in the same culture. On the other hand, there are universal aspects of social behaviour, found in all cultures. This is important for our present purposes, because patients must be taught behaviour which is appropriate in their sub-culture, and because a common social difficulty is dealing with people from other sub-cultural groups.

Several aspects of behaviour vary between cultures.

1. *Non-verbal signals*. Facial expressions are very similar in all cultures, though there are different rules about how freely they can be used. Gestures are much more variable, and each culture has a number of gestures with special meanings. The degree of proximity and use of bodily contact vary widely, as does the meaning of the *same* signal in these areas.

2. *Rules* for particular situations vary, e.g. buying and selling, at meals, giving presents. Barker and Wright (1954) showed that people are commonly aware of the rules for a large number of everyday situations in their culture – most of which would be somewhat different in another culture.

3. *Effect of ideas and language*. Different cultures categorise and label events, including social behaviour, in distinctive ways. In Britain we do not think much in terms of 'honour' or 'machismo', though some people think in terms of 'cool' and 'way out'. Ideals of behaviour also vary. In our society, it is normal to give help to those who depend on us, or to whom we have a professional duty, while in some societies recipients of help lose face and more importance is therefore attached to reciprocity.

4. *Social structure*. The relations between men and women, young and old, supervisor and subordinates, take different forms in different cultures, and within one culture are subject to changing climates of opinion. For example, we have recently moved towards greater equality of the sexes, and a more democratic-persuasive kind of leadership.

Intercultural communication can fail in several ways, which can be related to the problems of patients.

(i) The other person is rejected because his behaviour is seen as deviating from proper behaviour.

(ii) The other's signals are misunderstood. For example, bodily contact, common in Arab, Italian, or African cultures, is seen as a very intimate signal in Northern Europe and America.

(iii) The other's signals are misunderstood through not being aware of his ideas, ideals and cognitive world.

(iv) No attempt is made to accommodate, for example by shifting accent towards the other's accent. Attempts are made to impose rules as being the 'correct' ones.

CONCLUSION

In this chapter we have put forward the social skills model, looked at some of the many and complicated components of behaviour, and the rules governing their use. In the next chapter we shall turn to a discussion of how these skills are acquired in normal people, and describe the particular deficits of socially inadequate psychiatric patients.

References

ARGYLE, M. (1972) *The Psychology of Interpersonal Behaviour*, 2nd ed. Harmondsworth: Penguin.

ARGYLE, M. (1975) *Bodily Communication*. London: Methuen.

ARGYLE, M. (1976) Personality and social behaviour. In R. Harré (ed.), *Personality*. Oxford: Blackwell.

ARGYLE, M., ALKEMA, F. AND GILMOUR, R. (1972) The communication of friendly and hostile attitudes by verbal and non-verbal signals. *European Journal of Social Psychology*, 1, 385–402.

ARGYLE, M., INGHAM, R., ALKEMA, F. AND MCCALLIN, M. (1973) The different functions of gaze. *Semiotica*, 7, 19–32.

ARGYLE, M. AND KENDON, A. (1967) The experimental analysis of social performance. In L. Berkowitz (ed.) *Advances in Experimental Social Psychology*, vol. 3. New York: Academic Press.

ARGYLE, M., SALTER, V., NICHOLSON, H., WILLIAMS, M. AND BURGESS, P. (1970) The communication of inferior and superior attitudes by verbal and non-verbal signals. *British Journal of Social and Clinical Psychology*, 9, 221–31.

AUSTIN, J. L. (1962) *How to do things with words*. Oxford: Oxford University Press.

BARKER, R. G. AND WRIGHT, H. F. (1954) *Midwest and its Children: The Psychological Ecology of an American Town*. Evanston, Ill.: Row, Peterson.

BERNE, E. (1966) *Games People Play*. London: Deutsch.

BIRDWHISTELL, R. (1970) *Kinesics and Context*. Philadelphia: University of Pennsylvania Press.

DAVITZ, J. R. (1964) *The Communication of Emotional Meaning.* New York: McGraw-Hill.

EISLER, M. E., HERSEN, M., MILLER, P. M. AND BLANCHARD, E. B. (1975) Situational determinants of assertive behaviours. *Journal of Consulting and Clinical Psychology,* 43, 330–40.

EKMAN, P. (1971) Universals and cultural differences in facial expressions of emotion. *Nebraska Symposium on Motivation.*

EKMAN, P. AND FRIESEN, W. V. (1974) Nonverbal behavior and psychopathology. In R. J. Friedman and M. M. Katz (eds), *The Psychology of Depression: Contemporary Theory and Research.* Washington D.C.: Winston & Sons.

FLANDERS, N. A. (1970) *Analyzing Teaching Behavior.* Reading, Mass.: Addison-Wesley.

FOA, U. G. (1961) Convergences in the analysis of the structure of interpersonal behaviour. *Psychological Review,* 68, 341–53.

GERGEN, K. (1971) *The Concept of Self.* New York: Holt, Rinehart and Winston.

GOFFMAN, E. (1956) *The Presentation of Self in Everyday Life.* Edinburgh University Press.

GRAHAM, J. A. AND ARGYLE, M. (1975) A cross-cultural study of the communication of extra-verbal meaning by gestures. *International Journal of Psychology,* 1, 57–67.

JENNINGS, H. H. (1950) *Leadership and Isolation.* New York: Longmans, Green.

JONES, E. E. AND GERARD, H. B. (1967) *Foundations of Social Psychology.* New York: Wiley.

KENDON, A. (1967) Some functions of gaze direction in social interaction. *Acta Psychologica,* 26, 1–47.

KENDON, A. (1970) Movement coordination in social interaction: some examples considered. *Acta Psychologica,* 32, 1–25.

KENDON, A. (1972) Some relationships between body motion and speech. In A. Siegman and B. Pope (eds) *Studies in Dyadic Interaction.* Elmsford, N.Y.: Pergamon.

LEFCOURT, H. M. (1972) Recent developments in the study of locus of control. *Progress in Experimental Personality Research,* 6, 1–41.

LONGABAUGH, R. *et al.* (1966) The interactional world of the chronic schizophrenic patient. *Psychiatry,* 29, 78–99.

LORR, M. AND MCNAIR, D. M. (1965) Expansion of the interpersonal behavior circle. *Journal of Personality and Social Psychology,* 2, 813–30.

MEHRABIAN A. (1972) *Nonverbal Communication.* Chicago, Ill.: Aldine Atherton.

MELDMAN, M. J. (1967) Verbal behavior analysis of self-hyperattentionism. *Disorders of the Nervous System,* 28, 469–73.

MISCHEL, W. (1968) *Personality and Assessment.* New York: Wiley.

MOOS, R. H. (1969) Sources of variance in responses to questionnaires and in behaviour. *Journal of Abnormal Psychology,* 7, 405–12.

RUBIN, Z. (1973) *Liking and Loving.* New York: Holt, Rinehart & Winston.

SARBIN, T. R. AND JONES, D. S. (1956) An experimental analysis of role behavior. *Journal of Abnormal and Social Psychology*, 51, 236–41.

SCHEFLEN, A. E. (1965) *Stream and Structure of Communicational Behavior*. Commonwealth of Pennsylvania: Eastern Pennsylvania Psychiatric Institute.

SISSONS, M. (1970) The psychology of social class. In *Money, Wealth and Class*. London: Open University Press.

TURNER, R. H. (1956) Role-taking, role standpoint, and reference-group behavior. *American Journal of Sociology*, 61, 316–28.

3 Development and deficiency in social skills: a review of the evidence

Introduction

The social skills model put forward in the previous chapter provides a general framework for considering the complex rules underlying normal social behaviour, and we have suggested that many psychiatric patients lack these skills. This chapter will be concerned with some of the important practical questions raised by this general proposition. For example, how are social skills acquired and why do some people fail to acquire them? What do we mean when we say someone is socially unskilled or socially inadequate? Inadequate by whose standards? Do people agree on what constitutes social inadequacy? Which elements of behaviour have most influence on judgments of social skill? How many patients report difficulty in social situations or are behaviourally unskilled? What sorts of people are they most likely to be? What sorts of situations cause the most difficulty? How many 'normal' people are also inadequate?

This chapter will attempt to bring together what is known in order to answer some of these questions; others cannot yet be answered, or can be answered only partially, since very little work has been carried out on the problems of definition and prevalence. Because of this we shall draw extensively on two studies done by the authors, the first a survey of social inadequacy in psychiatric outpatients, and the second a survey of reported social difficulty in a non-psychiatric population, namely university students (Bryant *et al.* 1976; Bryant and Trower 1974). At the end of the chapter a few profiles of socially inadequate patients who have received social skills training will be described in order to put research findings in the context of real problems.

'Aetiology' of social inadequacy

The social skills model advanced in chapter 2 assumes that skills are acquired through various forms of learning, such as imitation, reinforcement and instruction, and through exposure to a wide range of environmental opportunities, and to skilled models such as parents, siblings, relatives, peers and others. It follows that failure to acquire them would occur through a dearth of either skilled models or social opportunities, though in practice it is not possible to separate these two influences. Despite the enormous quantity of research into socialisation in the child, few studies have looked specifically at the processes through which children mature into socially skilled adults or fail to do so.

PARENTS

Most research concerned with parent–child relationships has emphasised the development of emotional bonds rather than the acquisition of social skills. From the standpoint of social skills, the earliest environment and the first models available to the infant are the parents. What evidence is there that the social competence of parents is causally related to that of their children? Some studies suggest that warm, loving and positive parental relationships lead to more friendly, cooperative and attentive behaviour in the child (Schaefer and Bayley 1963), and it is possible that the child acquires this behaviour partly through imitation. Other explanations, such as genetic influences, are also possible; furthermore, the eliciting of warm responses from the parents may be related to the child's own disposition. One study of maladjusted individuals found that the mother's own cognitive/coping skills appeared to be more relevant for adjustment than her emotional warmth (Siegelman, Block, Block and von der Lippe 1970). A recent study in the United States by Sherman and Farina (1974) has shown that socially inadequate male college students were more likely than adequate students to have socially inadequate mothers, which the authors interpreted as supporting the idea of acquiring skills through imitation of the parents, although a genetic explanation was also possible. Since the students were all men, it is a pity that fathers were not included in the study. It may be noted in passing that fathers are conspicuous by their absence from most research concerned with parent–child relationships.

As well as providing models for their children, parents instruct them in proper behaviour, reinforcing appropriate and discouraging inappropriate behaviour. Instructions may often be quite explicit, revealing the parents' underlying grasp of social rules; for example, commands such as 'Look at me when I am talking to you', 'Don't interrupt', 'Say hello' are all very specific attempts to instill, in this case, appropriate looking, meshing and greeting behaviours. It is probable that socially unskilled parents will be less accurate in their perceptions of what is appropriate, and therefore less likely to instigate and reinforce skilled responses in their children.

Studies of the acquisition of sex-typed behaviour suggest that the processes of imitation and reinforcement may not be as simple as they are often thought to be. It has been assumed that children learn the skills appropriate to their sex through parental reinforcement and identification with (imitation of) the same sex parent. However, in a comprehensive review of the evidence, Maccoby and Jacklin (1975) came to the conclusion that this was an insufficient explanation. While parents differentiate between behaviour considered appropriate for boys and girls, they do not necessarily reflect this in their actions, and there are important areas of sex-differentiated behaviour where parental sanctions and encouragement seem to play only a very minor role. For example, aggressive behaviour appears to be discouraged, and autonomous, independent behaviour encouraged, equally in children of both sexes. Similarly, there is little evidence to support the idea that children selectively imitate the same-sex parent.

Maccoby and Jacklin suggest that while direct reinforcement and simple imitation are clearly involved, they serve to provide, along with other observations, a potential range of behaviours for both boys and girls, which only become differentiated as the child gradually develops the cognitive ability to induce rules from his observations. In other words, 'he gradually develops concepts of "masculinity" and "femininity", and when he has understood what his own sex is he attempts to match his behaviour to his conceptions'. If this is so, it is probably true for the acquisition of skills required for other social roles such as friend, enemy, schoolchild, senior, junior and so on.

SIBLINGS

Most children are reared in families containing siblings, and the family structure itself provides particular modelling and environmental opportunities, depending on the child's position in the birth order and the spacing and sex of siblings. Some of the implications of family structure will be discussed later in this chapter. Although it is obvious in one sense that the experience of, say, the youngest child of a large, dense family will be different from that of the eldest, and both different from that of an only child, not very much is known about how these experiences relate to later social skills. Later born children have been found to be more socially outgoing and stronger on measures of sympathy than first-born and only children, and later born boys and girls to be less submissive to authority (Sampson 1965), but the processes involved are not clear.

PEERS

In later childhood and adolescence much of the time is spent with peers, and numerous studies have shown that children's groups have norms of their own to which individuals learn to conform. It has also been shown that children use social techniques such as imitation to gain admission to groups (Phillips, Shenter and Revitz 1951). Peer groups provide models for imitation, and also opportunities for learning to influence others and so on, but very little is known about whether behaviour patterns established in early childhood are changed or rather reinforced by these experiences. It is reasonable to suppose that all children will have some peers who are socially skilled, which suggests that the mere availability of skilled models is not enough to ensure successful imitation. Previous experience with siblings may well be helpful in learning to get on with peers, but this has not been demonstrated.

Environmental factors, in which chance may play a large part, will in turn be tempered by the preferences of the individual and also by his ability to capitalise on the available opportunities.

ATTITUDES TO THE ENVIRONMENT

A number of writers have been interested in attitudes to the environment in relation to competence (Rotter 1966; Lefcourt 1966). Rotter has devised a scale of the 'locus of control' which classifies people into 'internal controllers' who feel in control of the environment and 'external controllers' who feel controlled by it. We have already commented on the importance of control as a dimension of social skills, and the inadequate patients in our outpatient survey were characterised by their inability to control and manage the situation they were in.

We know very little about how such attitudes are acquired, but one suggestion has been that contingent reinforcement – the timing by the mother of her responses to the infant so that he can become aware of the consequences of his behaviour – enables the child to acquire the belief that his actions can control the environment in the way he wants them to (Lewis and Goldberg 1969). Some mothers may be more sensitive to this than others. There is also some evidence that birth order is influential (p. 60). It is possible, although this can only be speculation, that early feelings of helpessness in social situations are related to later social inadequacy.

This could also be relevant to certain aspects of depression. Feelings of powerlessness to control the environment are common among patients with reactive depressions, and this has led to the suggestion that some depressions arc similar in form and origins to the phenomenon of learned helplessness in animals (Seligman 1974). Animals who have previously been exposed to inescapable shock are unable, under subsequent conditions of escapable shock, to learn avoidance behaviour, and they submit passively. Seligman suggests that the depressed patient has learned that he cannot control those elements of his life that relieve suffering or bring gratification, and therefore believes he is helpless. While rather unspecific about how this may arise, he suggests that it may be the result of a life-time's experience of situations in which the individual has been relatively devoid of mastery. This explanation, however, presupposes a remarkable, and perhaps rather improbable, constancy in environmental experiences. It is nevertheless interesting to speculate that repeated failures to master situations may occur not only through early established predisposing attitudes but also through inadequate social skills.

EFFECTS OF DEPRIVATION

The understanding of normal development can be enhanced by considering what happens to children brought up in 'abnormal' environments, and much interest has been shown in children reared under conditions of deprivation, such as those in institutions, in broken homes or in families with disrupted family relationships. The work in this field has been comprehensively reviewed by Rutter (1972).

Rutter concluded that privation or poverty of stimulation, such as that found in child-care institutions, has little effect on long-term emotional and behavioural adjustment, but can have negative consequences for cognitive development, and also that it is the distinctiveness and meaningfulness of the stimuli which are more important than the absolute level of stimulation.

Deprivation involving disturbed family relationships, on the other hand, seems to have bad consequences for emotional and behavioural adjustment but a negligible effect on cognitive development. Rutter distinguishes between the disruption of bonds (through death and divorce or separation) and the distortion of relationships (through discord, quarrelling and lack of warmth and affection). Results of studies reported by Rutter show that antisocial behaviour in children is associated with parental discord *per se*, either with or without break-up (divorce or separation), but not with the break-up of the home through death. In other words, what appears to be important is not the disintegration of the home but the discord within it.

It is possible that children in discordant families become antisocial, not so much because of emotional disturbance due to the breakup of parental relationships, but rather because they are following a deviant parental model of behaviour. Rutter argues that this is unlikely because the adverse effects of a poor parental marriage are ameliorated if the child manages to maintain a good relationship with one parent. However, this need not be inconsistent with the model hypothesis, since the good relationship implies that at least one parent is successfully interacting with the child, thereby providing a good model in this respect for the child to imitate.

Although Rutter was mainly concerned with antisocial or delinquent behaviour as opposed to social inadequacy, retrospective evidence from our outpatient study indicates that many of the inadequate patients also had parents who were probably bad models. We found that 42 per cent of inadequate patients came from distorted families, in the sense either that one or both parents were absent from home or themselves mentally ill or that they were described as being cold, harsh, tyrannical, critical, withdrawn and so on. (In an earlier study of ours, all but two out of sixteen inadequate patients had some family disturbance of this kind.) However, a similar proportion of the *adequate* patients (43 per cent) in the outpatient survey also came from such families, which would suggest that any association between social incompetence in parents and children is not a simple one, and that other factors may intervene which mitigate its effects. Perhaps the adequate patients were the ones who maintained a good relationship with one parent. Rutter mentions other factors modifying long-term effects, such as the age or temperament of the child, opportunities to develop attachments with other adults, and duration of separation and privation.

It is generally assumed that disruptive parental relationships lead to disturbance in the child, rather than the other way about. It is possible, however, that the arrival of a child in the family, and above all a difficult child, may itself become a source of discord and conflict leading to a deterioration in the parental relationship, as may the closeness of the child to one parent and not the other.

GENETIC INFLUENCES

Although the social skills model assumes the acquisition of skills through learning, it is probable that genetic influences are also active. This is not the place for a review of the nature/nurture controversy, and it must suffice to say that opinion has ranged in the past from the extremes of development seen as an orderly unfolding of inherent capacities to the explanation of all behaviour solely as a function of environmental learning. More recently psychologists have profitably abandoned these extreme positions, and their studies suggest that both innate and environmental factors play their part in the acquisition of social behaviour.

Recent studies of mother–infant relationships in particular have recognised the reciprocal nature of social interaction, and have pointed out that the individuality of the infant affects the mother's behaviour as well as the mother's behaviour affecting the infant (Bell 1968; Rheingold 1968; Schaffer 1971). It is probable, therefore, that from a very early age the innate predispositions of the child actively influence the sorts of experience he has.

COGNITIVE ABILITIES

The social skills model requires cognitive abilities for processing information, for making inferences about the consequences of courses of action, for taking the role of the other person, and so on. Developmental psychologists have long been concerned with how and at what ages these abilities develop. The most well-known is probably Piaget, who has claimed that children develop in a series of stages and that certain abilities are impossible if the child has not reached the appropriate stage. Some of his views have been questioned by Bryant, who has shown that some abilities occur at much younger ages than Piaget postulated – for example, the ability to make logical inferences, which has been demonstrated in children as young as three and four years instead of seven years as Piaget claimed (Bryant 1974).

Of particular relevance to social skills is the ability to perceive the world from another person's point of view. Piaget claims that young children under seven years are 'egocentric' and that a complete comprehension of another person's perspective does not occur until nine years. However, Borke (1975) has shown that, provided the task is made age-appropriate, children as young as three years can succeed on perceptual role-taking tasks. She comments: 'If one accepts the premise that the capacity to understand another person's perspective is a basic component of empathy, understanding is already present in children as young as three and four years of age.'

Although we did not specifically test their role-taking ability, the inadequate patients in our outpatient survey were found to show very little interest in the other person. Feffer and Suchotliff (1966) found that people who did well in a role-taking test also did well in a test of social interaction, and it is likely that the inability to take the role of the other is related to social inadequacy.

It has also been shown to be related to chronic delinquency in boys of ten and eleven years (Chandler 1973).

Although the processes are not clear, it is generally accepted that cognitive abilities occur through the combined influence of innate ability and environmental experience. The deprivation studies already mentioned show that an unstimulating environment, and in particular undifferentiated stimulation which lacks meaning with regard to the child's own responses, can adversely affect the development of cognitive abilities. Most of these studies have been concerned with language development and scholastic attainment rather than, for example, with perspective taking or problem solving abilities.

Parents who lack empathic or problem solving skills may contribute to limited growth of these and other skills in their children. If they are unable to put themselves in the child's position they may be insensitive to the child's responses and therefore provide poor stimulation of all kinds. If they resort to quarrelling to cope with their problems, they will provide a demonstration of poor, limited and inflexible problem solving skills for the child to imitate. It has not been demonstrated that this happens, but it seems a plausible hypothesis which warrants investigation.

CONCLUSIONS

It would seem from much of the research already mentioned that the development of social skills starts at a very early age, and that most of the basic 'ingredients' of the social skills model are probably already present in very young children of pre-school age. Clearly maturation also plays a part, since the complex interplay of verbal and non-verbal signals can only be synchronised as language advances, and the specific rules pertaining to particular situations can only be learned as these situations arise for the growing child. Despite the tantalising links which research findings offer concerning the quality of parent-child relationships and environmental experiences and the development of social skills, we can still only speculate on why some adults end up socially inadequate and others do not. One reason for this is that a great deal of experimental work is concerned with laboratory tasks involving objects rather than people or with scores on tests assumed to predict behaviour. The extent to which these results can be generalised to real life is not at all clear.

The idea that parental behaviour is influential in the development of psychiatric disorders is fundamental to psychiatric theory and practice. Interest has mainly been focussed, however, on emotionally disturbing factors in the parent–child relationship, such as conflict, dominance, excessive criticism, rejection and so on. These qualities can themselves be interpreted as socially unskilled responses to the child, and the social skills model provides an alternative theory about the nature of the role played by parents in the aetiology of psychopathology. As Sherman and Farina (1974) concluded in their study of college students and their mothers: 'The early patterns established in the home by skilled or unskilled parents may be of critical importance' (p. 330).

Although it seems likely that at least the rudiments of social skills develop or fail to develop in early childhood, Clarke and Clarke (1972) have warned against assuming that early experience will necessarily predetermine the course of later development and 'make or mar the child'. They point out that the correlations found in longitudinal studies of, for example, intelligence, personality and academic achievement, are not very high, and while they may indicate some consistency they also indicate considerable change. Furthermore, it is now generally acknowledged that change from extremely adverse environments into better ones tends to be followed by desirable changes in behavioural characteristics. It is nevertheless possible that if inadequate social skills for controlling the behaviour of others are acquired in the early years, they may serve to reduce both the range of subsequent experiences and the quality of learning that can occur in them.

The nature of social inadequacy

From the point of view of clinical practice a clear definition of social inadequacy is needed. How is it to be defined, and, following from this, how is it to be measured? These questions are easy to ask but unfortunately extremely difficult to answer, for a number of reasons which will be briefly discussed.

1. Social inadequacy is a phenomenon derived from social norms, and it suffers the inevitable difficulties of subjectivity and imprecise definition. The problem is, how far do people agree on what is socially appropriate behaviour? If they do not agree, whose

standards should be adopted? Furthermore, are patterns the same for everybody, or do they vary with the age, sex, social class, and so on, of either the subject or judge? We know that patterns of non-verbal communication vary widely from culture to culture, and we have some evidence, as we shall see, that different standards are adopted for two basic groups in our society, men and women.

2. Social inadequacy has come to mean different things in psychiatry. In one sense all psychiatric disorders are manifestations *to others* of behaviour which is then judged *by others* to be abnormal, and which, subsequently, may be seen as constituting one of a cluster of behaviours which is given a particular diagnostic label. In other words, behaviour is abnormal because it occurs in a *social* context requiring social norms to which it does not conform. Indeed, the mere verbal claim to a disturbed mental state without accompanying behavioural abnormality may well be doubted. This approach, however, is clearly too wide to be of use, and we can start by confining the problem to the particular behaviours used in communication and to the specific rules of social situations.

This still leaves us, however, with a very wide area. Concepts of social competence crop up in many branches of psychiatry. They are most explicitly recognised in 'cure' and rehabilitation, where the assessment of an individual's fitness to return to family and society has resulted in a number of measures of social competence – unfortunately using many different criteria. In subnormality, social skills may include personal management such as ability to do up buttons, tie shoe laces, use a knife and fork, count and handle money. In rehabilitation of hospitalised patients, the term social incompetence is often used to refer to the inability to cope with a limited range of social situations essential to day-to-day life, such as shopping, going on buses, regular time keeping at work, and so on. The term is also used to describe the gross social withdrawal exhibited by institutionalised schizophrenic patients whose social behaviour appears to be almost totally suspended, even to the extent of neglect of personal appearance and double incontinence. The limited expectations for such patients are reflected in rating scales designed for their assessment. Ratings of verbal behaviour, for example, may range from muteness to the simple ability to answer questions coherently (Harris *et al.* 1967).

This sort of behaviour bears little resemblance to the relatively sophisticated social skills discussed in the previous chapter, and the programme of social skills training provided in the second half of this book is not intended to deal with it. This is not to say that a social behavioural approach to such problems is ruled out, but that it would require a different technique and more limited goals. For this reason psychotic and brain damaged patients will be excluded from consideration in the rest of this chapter, along with the special problem of addiction to alcohol or drugs (in which organic deterioration may affect behaviour). This leaves us with the large area of anxiety states, reactive depressions and personality disorders which constitute about two-thirds of outpatient diagnoses, in which behaviour deficits are less gross, and for which social therapies such as social skills training may be rather more appropriate.

3. There is no psychiatric diagnostic category which clearly fits the inadequate individual, and social inadequacy cuts across diagnoses. It is not uncommon in case notes to see such phrases as 'social difficulty' appended to conventional diagnoses of depression, anxiety states and personality disorders. Traditionally, psychiatrists have mainly confined their interest to social inadequacy as a personality type, emphasising enduring traits such as weakness, timidity, anxiety and passive attitudes. Perhaps the nearest to our behavioural definition are the 'inadequate' and 'passive' personality types subsumed under aesthenic personality in the *International Classification of Diseases*, but these are very briefly and generally described, and the section of the *I.C.D.* concerned with personality disorders has itself come under recent criticism (Shepherd and Sartorius 1974). Indeed, the whole area of abnormal personality is fraught with problems common to all typologies. They are not clearly separate classes, but abstractions, typical in an ideal but not necessarily in a statistical sense, and although some features may be prominent in a 'type' they often merge with other types. It is not surprising that a very poor level of agreement has been reached between psychiatrists in assigning individuals to personality types (Zubin 1967).

It was for this reason that we carried out a survey of social inadequacy among psychiatric outpatients to try to provide an empirical definition, and also to investigate the clinical and social factors associated with it. Since this survey will be mentioned in some detail, a brief description of its methods is given.

THE OUTPATIENT SURVEY

The survey was carried out in a 14-bed psychiatric unit attached to a general hospital; it was chosen because it provided a single service which dealt with nearly all the referrals from the area. All patients attending this clinic over a six-month period who were diagnosed as having neuroses and personality disorders and who were aged 18–49 comprised the basic survey population.

Information on each patient was obtained from a clinical interview with the clinic psychiatrist, and from psychometric tests and other questionnaires. In addition, each patient took part in an eight-minute structured social situation test involving conversation with a stranger, and their behaviour was rated by two psychologists (one male, one female). Ratings of social inadequacy were also made by the clinic psychiatrist from the behaviour he observed in the clinical interview, and by a second psychiatrist who merely read the case notes, and never saw the patient.

BEHAVIOURAL CHARACTERISTICS OF INADEQUATE PATIENTS

Part of the analysis of the outpatient survey took the form of comparing a group of adequate patients (those whom all four raters had agreed were socially skilled) with a group of inadequate patients (whom all agreed were socially unskilled) on elements of behaviour. Behaviour was rated by the two psychologists on two dimensions: (a) the severity of the deficit (from normal to extremely abnormal) and (b) the direction of the deficit (from too much of the behaviour to too little of it).

The results, given in table 3.1, showed the inadequate patients to be markedly inferior to the adequate patients on most of the twenty-four behavioural elements, and also on six of seven overall judgments of such qualities as warmth, assertiveness, control. Furthermore, almost all of this deficit was in the direction of too little use of behaviour rather than too much.

In detail, it was shown in conversation that the inadequate patients showed little variation in facial expression, which was predominantly blank and unsmiling, or in posture, which was predominantly 'closed' and inflexible, and they looked very little at the other person. They were not, however, distinguished from adequate patients by their general appearance. They spoke too

Table 3.1   Comparison of Group i (adequate) and Group v (inadequate) on the Elms Rating Scale

	Group i		Group v		
	Mean	*S.D.*	*Mean*	*S.D.*	P
Non-verbal : voice					
Volume	1·42	0·50	2·20	0·86	·001
Tone	1·50	0·65	2·30	0·94	·001
Clarity	1·19	0·40	2·20	1·08	·001
Speed	1·19	0·49	2.07	1·03	·001
Non-verbal : body					
Facial expression	1·50	0·71	2·93	1·10	·001
Gaze	1·36	0·76	2·07	1·28	·05
Posture	1·81	0·80	2·68	1·11	·01
Verbal : form					
Length	1·62	0·70	2·80	1·08	·001
Spontaneity	1·13	0·68	2·33	1·18	·001
Control	1·96	0·72	2·47	1·13	
Continuity	1·35	0·49	2·80	1·01	·001
Silences	1·96	0·72	3·32	0·82	·001
Hesitations	1·19	0·40	1·60	0·99	
Handing over	1·92	0·53	3·07	0·88	·001
Taking up	1·54	0·58	1·93	0·88	
Verbal : content					
Topics	1·46	0·71	3·07	0·88	·001
Interest in other	1·58	0·64	2·53	0·99	·001
Interest in self	1·27	0·60	2·47	0·92	·001
Feeling talk	1·46	0·65	2·47	0·92	·001
Total score on E.R.S.	10.31	5.84	30·60	8·05	·001

(Test of significance : t test for independent samples.)

softly, indistinctly and slowly, and in a flat and monotonous tone. Their speech lacked continuity and was punctuated with too many silences; they failed to hand over or take up the conversation, and generally did little or nothing to control the interaction, leaving the other person to make all the moves. They chose stereotyped and dull topics and showed little interest in the other person On the only two elements in which they 'over-performed', i.e. used the behaviour too much, which were 'interest in self' and 'feeling talk' (disclosure of their own emotions and mood), they tended to allow their personal problems and mood to intrude inappropriately into the conversion. They were no worse than adequate patients in the frequency of hesitations, interruptions and disagreements.

These behavioural deficits resulted in the inadequate patients being rated as significantly more cold, non-assertive, socially anxious, sad, unrewarding and uncontrolling than the socially skilled patients. On psychometric tests they emerged as significantly less dominant, sociable and self-accepting, and as significantly more introverted, but not more neurotic (see table 3.2).

Table 3.2 Comparison of Group i (adequate) and Group v (inadequate) on 'Personality' characteristics

	Group i		Group v		P
	Mean	S.D.	Mean	S.D.	
E.P.I.					
Neuroticism	15·69	5·07	17·79	4·64	
Extroversion	13·04	2·74	10·07	4·14	·01
Lie score	2·65	1·30	2·64	1·60	
C.P.I.					
Dominance	22·19	8·16	16·36	4·67	·02
Sociability	20·08	6·17	14·50	3·23	·01
Social presence	27·96	7·29	23·43	6·11	
Capacity for status	14·42	5·51	11·21	2·52	·05
Self-acceptance	18·08	4·43	14·57	4·20	·02
Previous personality					
Mixing in adolescence	1.15	0·37	2·47	1·19	·001
Sexual adjustment in adolescence	1·15	0·37	2·07	1·33	·01
Adjectives†					
Warm/cold	7·12	1·14	4·73	1·10	·001
Aggressive/*non-aggressive*	6·35	1·74	7·20	1·70	
Assertive/*non-assertive*	5·09	0·92	7·17	1·64	·001
Poised/socially anxious	5·88	1·66	4·40	2·13	·02
Happy/*sad*	5·85	1··32	7·80	0·94	·001
Rewarding/*unrewarding*	5·09	1·66	7·86	2·13	·001
Controlling/uncontrolling	6·88	1·34	4·47	1·41	·001

(† Poles in italics scored high.)
(Test of significance: t for independent samples.)

It is probably true to say that the sort of picture conjured up by this list of failings would fit many people's stereotype of an inadequate person. Such people, unfortunately, are often seen as basically submissive, which has led, as we shall see in chapter 5, to a great interest in training people to be more assertive. It is probably no coincidence that much of this work has been initiated in the U.S.A. where, as far as one can make generalisations of national characteristics, a high premium is placed on assertive and dominant styles of behaviour. This work has tended to neglect positive aspects of behaviour which can communicate warmth and empathy, factors at least as important to successful social interaction as assertiveness, if not more so. The inadequate patients described above were found to be not only less assertive and controlling but also less warm and rewarding.

Evidence for the importance of both rewarding and assertive behaviour was also provided by another group of patients in the outpatient study. These were patients about whom the four raters were equally divided in their ratings of social inadequacy. The behaviour of these patients was less often and less heavily marked down, but when it was it was because of over-use of behaviour. They tended to speak too loudly for too much of the time, and too much about themselves, to be too controlling and to treat the other person as an audience rather than an individual. They were rated as somewhat more aggressive and assertive than the adequate patients, but almost as cold and unrewarding as the inadequate patients.

The fact that the raters could not agree on whether this pattern of behaviour was inadequate suggests that it is more ambiguous in the message it carries. Such people can probably get by in social situations in the sense that they can participate actively, even if they are not very popular, and they may avoid isolation through their own insensitivity to the reactions of others and their ability to manipulate people.

Again, the two qualities found to correlate most highly with social skill were rewardingness ($\cdot78$) and control ($\cdot70$), two factors which have persistently emerged in many studies of group behaviour. They can be seen as constituting two basic subgroups of social skill which can be conceptually distinguished and which serve two distinct, although interrelated, purposes.

The first subgroup of skills, which may be called *facilitation skills*, have the purpose of maintaining social interactions at a rewarding level for all participants and encouraging (reinforcing) the behaviour and interest of the other. The elements of behaviour comprising them would be those described in chapter 2 which convey impressions of warmth, friendliness, sensitivity and like-ability.

The second subgroup, which may be called *controlling skills*, have the purpose of directing and controlling interactions. They would be comprised of the elements which are known to contribute to impressions of dominance, strength, control, assertiveness and so on.

We have some evidence from our outpatient study and from the work of others to support this distinction. In the outpatient study coldness was associated with one set of elements (e.g. silences, failure to hand over the conversation, dull expression and still posture), while unassertiveness was associated with a different set of elements (e.g. lack of initiative in conversation, lack of spontaneous speech, brief speech and soft volume). Eisler *et al.* (1973) also found assertiveness to be associated with voice, volume, length and spontaneity of speech. Mehrabian (1972) analysed the elements of social behaviour of student subjects and produced a three-dimensional scheme: evaluation (like/dislike), potency (dominant/submissive) and responsiveness (high activity). Responsiveness has not, however, been replicated by other investigators.

The inadequate patients in the outpatient survey clearly lacked both sorts of skill, while the group about whom the raters disagreed failed mainly in controlling skills, in the sense that they over-used them and were seen to be very assertive and aggressive. The fact that they were also seen as cold and unrewarding would imply that their over-controlling behaviour overshadowed and negated their otherwise adequate facilitation skills. Indeed it is likely that both types of skill interact in a complex way, in that the ability to be warm and rewarding is itself an aspect of control, and the ability to share the management of an interaction is itself an aspect of rewardingness. The synthesis of these two skills is difficult to achieve; some studies suggest that it may be achieved by good leaders through the use of democratic-persuasive styles.

AGREEMENT BETWEEN JUDGES

One aim of the outpatient survey was to investigate the degree of consensus between psychologists and psychiatrists, with their rather different professional backgrounds, in identifying patients who lacked social skills. The interrater reliability between all four raters was calculated and yielded a correlation coefficient of 0·76. This coefficient was statistically significant and indicates a reasonable level of agreement. This was despite the fact that the raters arrived at their judgments from different information about the patient, and that prior discussion with the clinic psychiatrist about the precise aims of the survey was deliberately avoided. These four raters comprised a very limited and specialised sample of raters, and their agreement cannot necessarily be taken as representative of the community at large.

In making their judgments of social inadequacy the psychiatrists were asked to do something which was not part of their normal clinical practice. While psychiatrists are trained to observe behaviour, they do this normally in order to make inferences about underlying psychic states and to arrive at a diagnosis, and it will be shown later in this chapter that social inadequacy was not closely related to diagnosis. It is unlikely, therefore, that most psychiatrists will identify the problem of social inadequacy using normal procedures, and it is partly for this reason that standard assessment procedures will be outlined in the second half of this book (p. 133).

Clinical factors

SYMPTOMS AND DIAGNOSIS

While social withdrawal is commonly found in schizophrenic patients, there is very little evidence available on whether lack of social skill is associated with other diagnoses – although some writers have pointed to the interrelationship between anxiety, depression and social difficulties (e.g. Libet and Lewinsohn 1973). We know that some highly anxious people develop phobias to specific social situations, but some of them show no apparent lack of social skills. It is known also that the ability to cope with and enjoy social interactions can be temporarily disrupted by reactive depression. Depressed patients often wish to avoid others, and, indeed, while depressed may show similar behaviour to socially inadequate patients, but on alleviation of symptoms they return to normal. Some depressed patients also have symptoms of anxiety. In a recent study comparing social skills training with desensitisation, we found that a number of inadequate patients also had symptoms of anxiety and social phobia.

In our outpatient survey we found no overall relationship between social inadequacy and any of the clinical measures used, such as diagnosis, symptoms, length of illness and so on. Symptoms of depression and anxiety were as common in the adequate as the inadequate patients. There was, however, a suggestion that in men social inadequacy was related to depression. There was no evidence that social inadequacy was associated with a diagnosis of inadequate personality. Although the clinic psychiatrist used this diagnostic category, in only four instances did it coincide with his own judgments of social inadequacy; moreover, three of the patients in the adequate group were also diagnosed as inadequate personality.

It seems that diagnostic practice is not a very useful way of identifying patients who lack social skills. In particular, where a diagnosis of neurosis is made, it may take precedence over social difficulties, and we estimate that about half of socially inadequate patients may be 'lost' in this way.

'PRE-MORBID PERSONALITY'

The concept of social inadequacy implies some element of persisting poor adjustment. We are not concerned with the temporary disruption of skills due to the onset of psychiatric symptoms, but with enduring difficulties which probably precede them. Information of this kind – on what is commonly called 'pre-morbid personality' – is often routinely sought in clinical examinations. This information is usually expressed in terms of whether the patient was a 'happy child', a 'poor mixer', 'got on well with others', 'made friends easily', 'dated with the opposite sex', and so on. The question arises whether, in fact, social inadequacy is related to 'previous personality' or long established difficulties.

The inadequate patients reported having significantly more difficulty in mixing with others and in 'dating' the opposite sex in adolescence, and were judged by the clinic psychiatrist to have had social difficulties long before their 'illness'.

This provides some evidence that social inadequacy is a persistent state, and also, perhaps, that inadequate skills may not be felt to be a problem until adolescence, when children move towards a more independent and less organised life in which they must seek out sexual partners, friends and groups to belong to. It is possible that some preventive work could be done at the adolescent stage with social skills training to avoid later social isolation and perhaps psychiatric breakdown.

REPORTED DIFFICULTY IN SOCIAL SITUATIONS

It can be argued that inadequate social behaviour does not really constitute a problem unless it gives rise to feelings of difficulty in social situations. Individuals, happily, vary enormously in how they like to present and express themselves, and those who show unusual social behaviour but are otherwise socially at ease or happy may be accepted as eccentric rather than inadequate. Such people provide colour to our lives, and we are not suggesting that this behaviour should be eradicated. We are concerned with those who feel that things are wrong and want to change them. The question arises whether those whom others judge to be inadequate are also the people who report the most difficulty.

Difficulty in social situations was measured in the outpatient survey with the Social Situations Questionnaire (see p. 139). This questionnaire was also given to a random sample of second year university students in order to obtain some data on a normal group.

The inadequate patients reported more difficulty across a wider range of situations than the adequate patients, but both groups had considerably worse scores than the students. The adequate patients, however, reported less difficulty than a subgroup of 'high difficulty' students who were felt to have considerable social problems.

Situations most often found difficult were, as might be expected, those involving actively seeking contact with relative strangers, particularly of the opposite sex. The highest correlations with social inadequacy across all patients were: approaching others and making the first move in starting up a friendship (·51), going out with someone of the opposite sex (·48), being with people you don't know very well (·47), being in a group of the opposite sex (·46), going to parties (·41), and meeting strangers (·40). A similar pattern was also found for the students. Unlike the students, however, the inadequate patients often reported difficulty in relatively less demanding situations; for example, nearly half of the inadequate group had difficulty in using public transport, and a quarter in walking down the street and going into shops. This suggests a fairly generalised component of social anxiety.

Social factors

Examination of the social factors related to social inadequacy may help to show what sorts of people are most likely to be inadequate, and may also provide some clues about how it develops. Again, there is very little direct evidence about either of these points, and our outpatient study provides much of the existing information.

SEX

Much attention has been paid by psychologists to sex-linked social behaviour, and it is generally agreed that boys and girls show different behaviour patterns at a very early age. How this comes about is less clear, although imitation and reinforcement are both likely to be involved.

The behaviour of the inadequate patients in the outpatient survey would seem to depart from stereotypes of both male and female behaviour, in particular, qualities of independence and assertiveness for men and warmth and empathy for women. It might be expected, therefore, that inadequate patients would be equally drawn from men and women.

The results of the outpatient survey clearly showed that this was not so; 46 per cent of the men in the sample were judged to be socially inadequate compared with only 16 per cent of the women.

A closer look at the results revealed an interesting fact. The difference between men and women held for *overall* judgments of inadequacy but not for ratings of elements of behaviour or qualities. Women were judged by the two psychologists to be as cold, unassertive, unrewarding and uncontrolling as the men, and were found to have similar scores on the personality tests. Rather more surprisingly, they were also judged to perform as poorly as the men on the behavioural elements, which were rated according to their degree of inappropriateness to the situation. In other words, although the raters felt that the women performed inappropriately, they still did not rate them as inadequate. This provides clear evidence of a double standard being applied to men and women.

Not only did the women show the same behavioural defects as the men, but they also had the same long-standing difficulties in mixing and reported as much difficulty in social situations. If these difficulties were going unrecognised because of different standards being applied to women, this could be said to constitute a kind of 'enforced' social inadequacy, enforced through not being acknowledged – by society in general, and by psychiatry in particular, from which, ironically, they were seeking help.

In practical terms the implications for treatment are considerable. Social norms change, and many of the values underlying attitudes to women are themselves being questioned. This poses a dilemma: on the one hand, adherence to old standards may deny help to some women who could benefit from therapies such as social skills training; on the other hand, the adoption of a more progressive stance could result in new standards being imposed on some women which they (or their families) are not ready to accept and which may sever them even further from their own social environment. The implications are not just for assessment but also for the actual training – for example, how controlling and assertive should women be taught to be? It is easy to dodge this issue by saying that each patient must decide this for herself. However, it does not obviate the point that therapists do impose their own standards on their patients, and must confront the social and moral implications of what they are doing.

MARITAL STATE

Marriage is considered a natural and highly desirable state in our society, and great pressures are put on individuals to conform to this expectation. However, successful courtship and the establishment of a stable marital relationship require considerable interpersonal skills, and it might be expected that inadequate patients, many of whom are known to have had dating difficulties in adolescence, would find it hard to achieve. We would therefore predict that a disproportionate number of inadequate patients would be single.

The results of the outpatient survey showed this to be so for men but not for women. Almost all the inadequate men were single, although in the survey as a whole 60 per cent of the men were married. A likely explanation for the high number of single men is that the male skills needed for courtship are just those that socially inadequate men lack – skills of assertiveness and control in particular. A somewhat similar argument was put forward many years ago to explain the consistently found preponderance of unmarried male, but not female, schizophrenic patients (Ødegaard 1946).

In the case of women the explanation is probably less straight-forward. Women are required to take less initiative in courtship, and inadequate women would therefore be likely to encounter less difficulty than inadequate men. It is also possible that some women who resist social pressures to marry may be more socially competent than average.

SOCIAL CLASS

Links between social skills and social class have received little direct attention in the literature. The effects of social class on intellectual attainment, patterns of child rearing and patterns of language use have received more attention, and will be dealt with only briefly here. It has been claimed that middle class parents make less use of physical punishment and more use of love-oriented techniques than lower class parents, that they provide more opportunities for the child to learn basic problem-solving strategies which can generalise to future problem situations, that they place more emphasis on goal-directedness, and that middle class language patterns are more flexible and less context-bound, resulting in a greater scope for operating within a wide range of of alternatives (summarised in Bruner 1971).

Goal-directedness and the related cognitive ability to envis-age alternative solutions in the light of the perceived situation (problem-solving skills) are both central to the social skills model. It might be expected, therefore, in the light of research findings, that social class would be related to social inadequacy, in the sense that lower class individuals would be more likely to lack these skills. This was not found in the outpatient survey, although there was a trend towards more social class IV and V patients in the inadequate group.

Some may infer from the findings that the social skills model is itself a model of middle class social skills, although we believe the model to be entirely independent of culture. Spivack and Shure

(1974), discussing the same point in relation to their training programme for problem-solving skills, found that a high level of problem-solving skills was related to better social adjustment at all socio-economic levels. They concluded that 'the well adjusted individual irrespective of social class may be one who weighs the possibilities and decides . . . what action is most appropriate for him at a given moment'.

Particular patterns of use of non-verbal and verbal signals are culturally determined, and it is fairly obvious on purely subjective grounds that they vary between social classes. In as far as people largely mix with others from the same social level as themselves, these different patterns are neither better nor worse than each other, but simply 'normal' in their context, and it may be that different standards are unconsciously adopted in assessing them, in much the same way as they appear to be adopted for men and women. Difficulties might be encountered in situations of upward or downward mobility, and lower class jibing at 'toffee-nosed' middle class people or middle class resentment of the 'brash upstart' may well indicate that in such situations standards are confused. In the student survey we found that students from working class backgrounds – who were in a predominantly middle class milieu at Oxford University and who were by definition themselves upwardly mobile – reported significantly more difficulty in social situations than other students. This may suggest that in an unfamiliar social environment they were unsure how to behave, and felt that their customary behaviour was inappropriate.

BIRTH ORDER AND FAMILY SIZE

There have been many studies of the effects of birth order and family size which show these to be important social variables related to intelligence and achievement. Results have been less clear cut in the area of social behaviour, but Schachter (1964) found that, under conditions of stress, adults who were first-born or only children preferred the company of other people whereas later-born individuals preferred to cope alone. His explanation of this was that first-born children receive more rewards for affiliative behaviour from parents who are over-solicitous with their first child, and therefore develop strong habits of dependence. In support of Schachter, Hines (1973) found that first-born adults performed better under social reinforcement conditions, and

Johnson (1973) showed that they were more concerned with behaving in a socially desirable manner than later-born individuals.

A few studies have looked at the relationship of birth order to attitudes to the environment, or what has been termed the 'locus of control', which has already been mentioned (p. 41). Newhouse (1974) found that only children assumed credit for a lesser number of positive events than first-born or later-born children, while Crandall, Katkovsky and Crandall (1965), in a study of older children, found the same for both only children and first-born children.

The implications of all these findings for social inadequacy are not entirely clear. In as far as dependence on others suggests conciliatory rather than assertive behaviour, and negative attitudes to the environment suggest passivity, and both suggest anxiety in social situations, it might be expected that first-born and only children would be more likely to be socially inadequate than later-born children. There was some evidence from our outpatient survey that the inadequate patients tended to come from one- or two-child families, although this was not statistically significant. In the student survey it was found that significantly more of the students who reported the greatest difficulty in social situations also came from such families.

It should be pointed out, however, that the effects of birth order and family size have not been entirely consistent, and some studies done on young children rather than adults suggest that second- or later-born children show greater dependence than first-born children (McGurk and Lewis 1972; Waldrop and Bell 1964). The significance of the spacing of children was examined by Waldrop and Bell who found greater dependency in later-born children from large families with short intervals between siblings.

Explanations of the effects of birth order and family size have largely been environmental ones, such as parental treatment or opportunities for mixing with other children. However, Bell (1968) argues that there may be genetic factors operating, such as that the physiology of pregnancy and delivery is different for first- versus later-born children, and that second and later neonates show higher skin conductivity which is related to heightened arousal. He concludes that until the effects of these influences have been isolated, interpretations solely in terms of environmental experiences should be qualified.

The extent of social inadequacy

Having discussed what we know of social inadequacy in terms of behaviour and of social factors, we may now turn to a consideration of its extent. How many people are socially inadequate? Is this a common problem or a relatively rare one? As with most other aspects of the problem, there is very little evidence available from which these questions can be answered.

One of the aims of the outpatient survey was to investigate this, at least in a psychiatric population. Taking the most conservative estimate, that all four raters agreed in identifying the problem, one in six patients or 17 per cent were found to be socially inadequate (one in three of the men and one in eleven of the women). On a slightly less stringent criterion, that three out of the four raters agreed, these ratios are increased to one in four (one in two of the men and one in six of the women).

These results pertain only to diagnoses of neurosis and personality disorder. They represent between 9 and 15 per cent of the patients of *all* diagnoses aged 18–49 who attended the clinic during the six-month period, but this is almost certainly a considerable underestimate since many of the patients excluded from the study on grounds of diagnosis were also likely to have been inadequate, in particular many of the schizophrenic patients. Social inadequacy would appear to be a problem at least as common as other more traditional psychiatric problems, and three to five times as common, for example, as addictions, which comprised 3 per cent of the clinic attendances, or phobias, which have been estimated at some 3 per cent of psychiatric patients (Marks 1969).

In comparing frequencies it is important to consider how representative one sample population is of the total population. The extent to which the clinic in the outpatient survey was 'typical' of outpatient clinics in general is difficult to determine, owing to a scarcity both of official statistics and of other studies, and to the use of different sampling methods and diagnostic groupings. The clinic had a relatively low referral rate, which suggests that it was unlikely to be providing a 'luxury' service for less disturbed people who would have avoided referral to psychiatric services in other areas. Comparisons with some other studies also suggest that the diagnostic frequencies found were not untypical (Gardiner *et al.* 1974; Kessel and Hassall 1971; Kessel and Shepherd, 1962).

The catchment area, however, although it was a mixed urban and rural one, did not contain any large cities.

These results tell us something about the extent of social inadequacy in a selected psychiatric population. They do not, however, provide any direct evidence on the extent of the problem in the normal population. The dividing line between people who seek psychiatric help for their difficulties and those who do not is a tenuous and sometimes arbitrary one, and there is every reason to believe that many people who do not become psychiatric patients have social difficulties. For instance, in our student survey – albeit a limited normal sample – we found that 9 per cent of the students reported considerable stress in common social situations, and although this is considerably less than the patient figure, it still represents a disturbingly high proportion.

Summary

In this chapter we have described the extent and nature of inadequate behaviour associated with other people's judgments of social inadequacy, and examined some of the available evidence on clinical and social factors associated with it, and on its possible 'aetiology'. What can we say in summary about the socially inadequate patient?

1. Socially inadequate patients of the sort we have been discussing will tend to show a particular style of behaviour. They will probably appear rather cold, unassertive and unrewarding to others, will show little expressive variation in face, voice and posture, will look rather infrequently at the other person, will make little effort to produce a spontaneous and interesting flow of speech, and will take little part in the management of conversations. Some of these behaviours may be difficult to assess in an initial clinical interview, which is usually controlled by the clinician, conducted using a question/answer technique, and in which the patient is not expected to show an equal personal interest in his interviewer.

2. On psychometric tests inadequate patients will tend to score rather higher than other patients on measures of introversion and social incompetence, but not neuroticism.

3. Clinically there may be little to distinguish the inadequate from the adequate patient, although a diagnosis of depression in

men may indicate a greater likelihood of inadequacy. In as far as previous personality and reports of social difficulty can be included as aspects of clinical state, inadequate patients will be likely to have had a history of poor mixing with others and of failure in dating, and to report considerable difficulty in a wide range of social situations, in particular those involving actively seeking contact with relative strangers, especially those of the opposite sex.

4. Men appear to be particularly 'at risk' for social inadequacy, and above all single men. However, we have seen that there is reason for caution in the acceptance of this finding, and therapists should be aware of the possible influences of their own preconceptions and values in the assessment of social inadequacy in women in particular.

5. Social class does not appear to be closely related to social inadequacy, although it may be relevant in certain situations where the individual is upwardly, or perhaps downwardly mobile, or is likely to be interacting with people of a different social class, for example, at work.

6. There is some suggestion that individuals who are only children or who come from small families may be more likely to be socially inadequate.

In considering these attributes, it should be remembered that they are not prerequisites of social inadequacy, but rather statistical averages which contain considerable individual variation. This means that any one individual will be unlikely to show all the behavioural deficits described, or all of the clinical and social attributes; furthermore, it is also possible that some of these factors may be present in adequate individuals. They should be considered rather as useful indicators of social inadequacy in following the assessment procedures described in the next section of this book.

Case histories

CASE 1

Mr P: aged 43, IQ 100.
Family history.   Father had skin trouble and phobia about dying. Mother dominant.

Personal history. Nervous, shy as a child; a stammerer. Did poorly at school, left at 14. Several unskilled jobs. No girl friends. Met a widow through marriage bureau, but panic set in when it came to marriage. Heterosexual but strongly inhibited. Occasional sex with prostitute.

Personality. Tends to busy himself at home. Always moody and anxious. Marked feeling of inferiority and inadequacy. Placid, dependent, marked obsessional traits.

On examination. Slight stammer, some facial twitching. Tense, anxious, mildly depressed. No suicidal ideas.

Social skills rating. Facially expressionless, rather stiff posture, tends to avert gaze, voice flat, poor handing over and taking up conversation, shows low interest in self and other. Rather cold, anxious and very unrewarding.

Social difficulty. Parties, pubs, dates, mixed groups, making close friends.

Clinical diagnosis. 'Personality disorder, immature, inadequate. Socially crippled'.

Previous health. From age 27, following death of father, depressed; insomnia for two years; thought he was mental. Had treatment from G.P. because of similar crises on and off since then.

CASE 2

Mrs D: aged 33, IQ 110.
Family history. Father died of cancer when she was aged three. Had some nervous trouble. Mother rather a tyrant. No siblings. Brought up by mother and an unmarried aunt. Felt unwanted.

Personal history. Left school at $17\frac{1}{2}$ with seven O-levels, but avoided A-level exam. Secretarial work, several jobs. Brought up away from influence of men. Aged 25 married. Husband a graduate, and feels inferior to him. Engaged for four years but no sexual intercourse until one year before marriage.

Personality. Described by G.P. as 'an introverted, schizoid personality'. Blushing aged 12–13 years. Never had any confidence. Never took the lead. Has always felt rather inadequate, and has difficulty mixing with people. No hobbies. Very conscious and ashamed of early breast development. Ashamed of sex since age ten.

Present problem. Referred by G.P. after separating from husband, some loss of sleep and appetite over last four weeks. Feels 'dead' – past depression. Never suicidal. Feels she cannot make contact with others. Distressed about possible divorce.

On examination. Smartly dressed. Did not look overtly depressed. Gave calm, rational account of problems, but at end burst into tears. Above average intelligence.

Social skills rating. Posture rather stiff, hand movements restless, shows low interest in other and self, poor handing over, speaks too long but very unassertive.

Social difficulty. Parties, mixed groups, entertaining, decisions affecting others, making close friends, keeping conversations going, talking about self.

Clinical diagnosis. 'Personality disorder; sexual difficulties; moderate depression'.

CASE 3

Mr B: aged 19, IQ 130.

Family history. Both parents Irish and working class. Father out a lot. Mother frequently hit children. No 'love in the family' and felt rejected. Has three brothers and two sisters.

Personal history. Shy and withdrawn at school, with few friends. Withdrew into studies and did extremely well. Attending university. Fear of others is now undermining his studies. Has one friend and never any girl friends.

Personality. Introverted, inhibited. Very low opinion of self and feels helpless to change things. Feels he is 'abnormal' and wants to be an ordinary person.

Present problem. Finds attending lectures and seminars almost impossible. Feels people are looking at him, feels very tense, cannot talk and cannot concentrate on what is being said. Avoids most lectures and spends much time alone in his room and ruminating on his failure.

On examination. Shoulder length hair which he uses to shield face. Head shaking and eyes watering. Dress not unusual for student. Reasonably forthcoming and insightful after a period.

Social skills rating. Marked gaze aversion and slumped posture. Talks in monosyllables, never initiates conversation, speaks too softly. Gives impression of extreme unassertiveness and anxiety.

Social difficulty. Starting conversations, being with girls, being with strangers.

Clinical diagnosis. 'Personality disorder with marked social phobia. Moderate depression'.

References

BELL, R. Q. (1968) A reinterpretation of the direction of effects in studies of socialization. *Psychological Review*, 75, 81–95.

BORKE, H. (1975) Piaget's mountains revisited: changes in the egocentric landscape. *Developmental Psychology*, 11, 240–3.

BRUNER, J. S. (1971) *The Relevance of Education.* London: Allen & Unwin.

BRYANT, B. M. AND TROWER, P. E. (1974) Social difficulty in a student sample. *British Journal of Educational Psychology*, 44, 13–21.

BRYANT, B. M., TROWER, P. E., YARDLEY, K., URBIETA, H. AND LETEMENDIA, F. (1976) A survey of social inadequacy among psychiatric outpatients. *Psychological Medicine*, 6, 101–112.

BRYANT, P. E. (1974) *Perception and Understanding in Young Children.* London: Methuen.

CHANDLER, M. J. (1973) Egocentrism and antisocial behaviour: the assessment and training of social perspective-taking skills. *Developmental Psychology*, 9, 326–32.

CLARKE, A. D. B. AND CLARKE, A. M. (1972) Consistency and variability in the growth of human characteristics. In Wall, W. D. and Varma, V. P. (eds) *Advances in Educational Psychology.* London: University Press.

CRANDALL, V. C., KATKOVSKY, W. AND CRANDALL, V. J. (1965) Children's beliefs in their own control of reinforcements in intellectual–academic achievement situations. *Child Development*, 36, 91–109.

EISLER, R. M., MILLER, P. M. AND HERSEN, M. (1973) Components of assertive behavior. *Journal of Clinical Psychology*, 29, 295–9.

FEFFER, M. AND SUCHOTLIFF, L. (1966) Decentering implications of social interactions. *Journal of Personality and Social Psychology*, 4, 415–22.

GARDINER, A. Q., PETERSEN, J. AND HALL, D. J. (1974) A survey of general practitioners' referrals to a psychiatric outpatient service. *British Journal of Psychiatry*, 124, 536–41.

GUNZBERG, H. C. (1964) The social competence of the severely mentally handicapped young adult. Paper read at the Conference of the International Committee for the Scientific Study of Mental Deficiency, Copenhagen.

68 Social skills and mental health

HARRIS, A. D., LETEMENDIA, F. J. J. AND WILLEMS, P. J. A. (1967) A rating scale of the mental state: for use in the chronic population of the psychiatric hospital. *British Journal of Psychiatry*, 113, 941–9.

HINES, G. H. (1973) Birth order and relative effectiveness of social and non-social reinforcers. *Perceptual and Motor Skills*, 36, 35–8.

JOHNSON, P. B. (1973) Birth order and Crowne-Marlowe Social Desirability scores. *Psychological Reports*, 32, 536.

KESSEL, N. AND HASSALL, C. (1971) Evaluation of the findings of the Plymouth Nuffield Clinic. *British Journal of Psychiatry*, 118, 305–12.

KESSEL, N. AND SHEPHERD, M. (1962) Neurosis in hospital and general practice. *Journal of Mental Science*, 108, 159–66.

LAZARUS, A. A. (1971) *Behavior Therapy and Beyond*. New York: McGraw-Hill.

LEFCOURT, H. M. (1966) Internal versus external control of reinforcement: a review. *Psychological Bulletin*, 65, 206–20.

LEWIS, M. AND GOLDBERG, S. (1969) Perceptual-cognitive development in infancy: a generalised expectancy model as a function of the mother–infant interaction. *Merrill-Palmer Quarterly*, 15, 81–100.

LIBET, J. M. AND LEWINSOHN, P. M. (1973) Concepts of social skills with special reference to the behavior of depressed persons. *Journal of Consulting and Clinical Psychology*, 40, 304–12.

MACCOBY, E. E. AND JACKLIN, C. N. (1975) *The Psychology of Sex Differences*. Stanford: University Press.

MCGURK, H. AND LEWIS, M. (1972) Birth order: a phenomenon in search of an explanation. *Developmental Psychology*, 7, 336

MARKS, I. M. (1969) *Fears and Phobias*. London: Heinemann.

MEHRABIAN, A. (1972) *Nonverbal Communication*. Chicago: Aldine-Atherton.

NEWHOUSE, R. C. (1974) Reinforcement-responsibility differences in birth order, grade level and sex of children in grades 4, 5 and 6. *Psychological Reports*, 34, 699–705.

ØDEGAARD, Ø.(1946) Marriage and mental disease. *Journal of Mental Science*, 92, 35.

PIAGET, J. AND INHELDER, B. (1956) *The Child's Conception of Space*. New York: W. W. Norton.

PHILLIPS, E. L., SHENKER, S. AND REVITZ, P. (1951) The assimilation of the new child into the group. *Psychiatry*, 14, 319–25.

RHEINGOLD, H. L. (1968) The social and socializing infant. In Goslin, D. A. (ed.) *Handbook of Socialization Theory and Research*. New York: Rand McNally.

ROTTER, J. (1966) Generalized expectancies for internal vs. external control of reinforcement. *Psychological Monographs: General and Applied*, whole number 609.

RUTTER, M. (1972) *Maternal Deprivation Reassessed*. Harmondsworth: Penguin.

SAMPSON, E. E. (1965) The study of ordinal position: antecedents and outcome. *Progress in Experimental Personality Research*, 2, 175–228.

Development and deficiency in social skills   69

SCHACHTER, S. (1964) Birth order and sociometric choice. *Journal of Abnormal and Social Psychology*, 68, 453–6.

SCHAEFER, E. S. AND BAYLEY, N. (1963) Maternal behaviour, child behaviour, and their intercorrelations from infancy to adolescence. *Monograph of Social Research in Child Development*, 82, No. 3.

SCHAFFER, H. R. (1971) *The Growth of Sociability*. Harmondsworth: Penguin.

SELIGMAN, M. E. P. (1974) Depression and learned helplessness. In Freedman, R. J. and Katz, M. (eds) *The Psychology of Depression: Contemporary Theory and Research*. Washington: Winston-Wiley.

SHEPHERD, M. AND SARTORIUS, N. (1974) Personality disorder and the International Classification of Diseases. *Psychological Medicine*, 4, 141–6.

SHERMAN, H. AND FARINA, A. (1974) Social adequacy of parents and children. *Journal of Abnormal Psychology*, 83, 327–30.

SIEGELMAN, E., BLOCK, J., BLOCK, J. H. AND LIPPE, H. VON DER (1970) Antecedents of optimal psychological development. *Journal of Consulting and Clinical Psychology*, 35, 283–9.

SPIVACK, G. AND SHURE, M. (1974) *Social Adjustment of Young Children*. San Francisco: Jossey-Bass.

WALDROP, M. AND BELL, R. W. (1964) Relation of preschool dependency behaviour to family size and density. *Child Development*, 35, 1187–95.

WEISBERG, P. (1963) Social and nonsocial conditioning of infant vocalizations. *Child Development*, 34, 377–88.

ZUBIN, J. (1967) The classification of the behavior disorders. *Annual Review of Psychology*, 18, 373–401.

4 Changing social behaviour

Introduction

How can social behaviour be changed? We have described some of the normal patterns and processes of social interaction, but in order to use this knowledge we need to develop ways of acquiring or modifying social behaviour. A great number of techniques for changing behaviour have been developed in recent years, and for convenience these may be grouped as follows: the first group may be termed *skills training*, which is aimed at changing social behaviour directly and derives mainly from experimental and particularly social psychology; the second includes the *dynamic techniques*, such as sensitivity training and psychotherapy, which aim to change relationships by means of awareness and insight; the third includes *milieu treatments*, where the total environment is planned along therapeutic lines; and the fourth may be termed *'symptom' treatments*, such as behaviour therapy and drugs which indirectly produce change by eradicating or suppressing disruptive symptoms. The main emphasis in this chapter and chapter 5 will be on the first group, with brief discussion of the others where relevant to the main theme.

Skills training

A number of principles of skill learning have been developed in laboratory settings and in applied fields such as industry and education, as well as mental health. We shall first describe these learning principles and their experimental basis, and then examine some of the more useful and successful applications.

PRINCIPLES OF SKILL ACQUISITION*

Implicit in the term 'training' is the notion of teaching people skills, and to do this we need to know about the best methods of acquiring skill. Experimental psychology has a long and respected history investigating the principles that govern skilled performance in both laboratory tasks and field settings. The bulk of this work has been on the learning and performance of perceptual and motor (or mechanical) skills (Fitts and Posner 1967; Legge 1970; Welford 1968). We have argued that the principles underlying skilled performance on these tasks can be applied to social behaviour, and that social interaction may be viewed as a form of skilled behaviour. This model has been described in chapter 2.

Many practitioners have drawn loosely upon the concept of 'social skills' in their clinical practice. Although the experimenta¹ research is complex and subject to constant changes in theory and method, it reveals some basic principles which have clear implications for treatment programmes based upon a model of training in social skills.

Practice
Practice makes perfect. The familiar proverb underlines that practice is essential in skills acquisition. Holding (1965) provides a succinct summary of the experimental work on practice in perceptual and motor skills. In the first place, practice is *necessary* for skills acquisition; but the amount needed will depend on the complexity of the skill to be acquired. To state this is to state the obvious to anyone who has attempted to hit a golf ball, drive a car or ride a bicycle. Of more interest are the conditions under which practice is most effective.

Crossman (1959) has demonstrated that there is a relationship between the amount of practice and the degree of skill, and that

---

* We have adopted the terminology of skills theory, but should point out that there are optional terms (sometimes used mistakenly), such as the following: 'role-playing' and 'behaviour rehearsal' for 'practice'; 'reinforcement' for 'feedback'; 'modelling' for 'demonstration', and 'instruction' and 'coaching' for 'guidance'.

even over several years people continue to improve with frequent practice. This contrasts with earlier beliefs that there are 'plateaus' in learning during which no improvement occurs. Skills learning is also seen as a gradual process, although in some instances of very simple skills, rapid acquisition can take place with a short period of practice. In tackling a complex skill should we practise the whole skill or only part of it? This depends on a number of factors. A more intelligent, capable individual, for instance, may master a skilled task by the 'whole' method, whereas a less capable person may need to progress bit by bit. But the most important factor is the nature of the task itself. With very complex tasks 'whole' learning is simply impossible as the techniques upon which the performance depends may not be in the subject's repertoire. Part learning is essential in these cases. In learning a very simple skill, on the other hand, part learning may be unnecessary and inefficient. In dividing a task into parts, it is important to select those parts which can be appropriately and easily combined into the whole. Practice on parts of a task which demand very different actions from the task as a whole is not likely to be very helpful. Nor is repetitive practice of small parts, as the effort involved is unlikely to be rewarded when the whole task is attempted. In devising a training programme for complex skills it is clearly important to subdivide the skills into the most appropriate component parts, bearing in mind these considerations.

Practice can be carried out frequently with short intervals between sessions or infrequently with longer intervals. This is technically known as the difference between *massed* and *spaced* practice. Massed practice generally leads to initial depression of performance and subsequent gains between trials. There seems to be little to differentiate the two methods in the long term, since both methods produce similar levels of improvement. In clinical situations, however, immediate improvement is generally desirable in order to keep the patient's motivation sufficiently high to persist, and this suggests that spaced practice might be of more value. Finally, practice can involve more than physically repeating a task or components of it. There is some evidence to indicate that silent rehearsal of activities, or mental practice, improves performance on skilled activities.

Feedback
Skills are not learned by practice alone. Although practice is

necessary to skills acquisition, it is not *sufficient*. In order to develop and improve skilled behaviour individuals need to have information about the consequences of their actions. For example, in throwing a ball at a target increased accuracy will only occur if the individual knows how close each attempt is. This is known as *knowledge of results* (Annett 1969). If all knowledge of results is artificially withheld from individuals attempting a skilled task – by preventing their seeing how close each throw is to the target, for example – then skilled performance does not improve. Thus, in addition to repeated practice, information must be fed back to the individual on his performance.

Information on success or failure can come in many ways. It may reside in the task itself and is then called *intrinsic feedback*. An example of such feedback is the muscular movements involved in throwing a ball. They will provide some information about the power in each throw which can be used in adjusting to subsequent throws. Alternatively, information can be supplied by factors external to the task and it is then called *extrinsic feedback* (sometimes also called 'augmented' or 'extra' feedback). An experimenter who tells each subject how close his throw is to the target is providing extrinsic feedback.

What is the relationship between intrinsic and extrinsic feedback and what combination is optimal for skills learning? Research has shown that extrinsic feedback will aid skilled performance. In a task in which subjects are required to pull a lever with a precise degree of pressure, a visual display plotting the accuracy of each attempt greatly enhances performance. But subjects do not always benefit from extrinsic feedback. This is illustrated by an experiment conducted by Goldstein and Rittenhouse (1954) on training gunners to hit aircraft in a simulator. If extrinsic feedback was given by a buzzer each time a target was hit, subjects showed immediate improvement. But as soon as the buzzer was withdrawn, performance deteriorated and subjects actually performed worse than a group who did not receive extrinsic feedback. It is clear that subjects may attend to extrinsic feedback at the expense of the feedback intrinsic in the task itself. This means that extrinsic feedback will be useful if it is programmed in such a way as to highlight rather than obscure intrinsic feedback (Holding 1965). Also, it should be faded out as subjects improve, to prevent them becoming dependent on this external source of information.

Another widely studied aspect is the optimal timing of feedback. Experiments on trial and error learning in animals show that feedback must be immediate to be effective. However, the role of feedback in human skills learning is more complex. Bilodeau and Bilodeau (1958), for example, have shown that human subjects can improve on a skilled task even when feedback is delayed up to twenty-four hours. Delay itself is thus not the significant factor in impaired performance. However, if another response intervenes between the response and its feedback, then skilled performance is markedly impaired. The intervention of other responses clearly prevents the subject from using the information to improve his performance, perhaps by muddling the relationship between the information from the response and that from the extrinsic feedback. Holding (1965) distinguishes between *concurrent* feedback, which is information provided during the task, and *terminal* feedback, which is information presented on its completion. Terminal feedback forces subjects to attend to the intrinsic cues in the task during its performance and presents information in a succinctly coded form at the end of the task. Verbal comments, for example, can be used as terminal feedback to present a considerable amount of information to subjects in a brief and succinct form. It seems that extrinsic feedback is most successful when given at the end of a response and presented in such a way as to highlight the intrinsic feedback in the task. Extrinsic feedback presented concurrently may produce initial improvements in performance but may also obscure the feedback in the task itself, resulting in poor skills acquisition in the longer term.

Demonstration

Demonstration plays an important role in learning complex tasks. It can take many forms. An instructor may simply tell subjects what to do, or he can demonstrate his own expertise. He might provide a film or videotape of others performing the task successfully. Or he may assign individuals to observe and imitate experts working on the job. What role does demonstration play in skills acquisition and what is the best way of demonstrating a task to ensure more successful skills acquisition?

Demonstration has three main functions. Firstly, it can draw attention to and magnify important components in a task. Thus a filmed sequence could be used to focus on a particular action in a complex skill and its importance can be underlined by slowing down the speed of the film and repeating the sequence – the 'action replay' effect. This may serve to direct the learner towards performing certain actions and not others. Secondly, the demonstration of a task serves to set a standard for future attempts. The subject is informed of the correct level of performance by means of the demonstration. Finally, demonstration serves as a basis for imitation. Recent work on imitation learning, or 'modelling', has shown that relatively complex human behaviour can be learned by observing and imitating others (Bandura 1969, 1971).

The most successful type of demonstration will depend to a large extent on the nature of the task. With simple tasks, extensive displays will not be necessary, and simple instruction may suffice. With more complex tasks, filmed or videotape demonstrations of components of the tasks can prove very beneficial. An important aspect of all demonstrations, however, is their integration into the task performance. Passive observation of a demonstration will be less effective than observation combined with active participation. Apart from preventing attention loss, participation ensures that the skill demonstrated is immediately translated into practice. This is likely to result in more effective learning. The opportunity for group involvement and discussion that accrues from demonstration has also been emphasised.

Many studies have investigated the effects of different types of models in imitation learning. This research has been concerned primarily with social behaviour in an experimental setting. The most effective model is generally one of high status with considerable power. Imitation is also more likely if more than one model is observed and if subjects perceive the model to be like themselves. Meichenbaum (1971) has shown that fearful subjects were more likely to imitate a model who appeared initially fearful but coped with her fear than one who showed no fear at all. This was particularly the case if the model verbalised her fears and her means of coping with them. In planning the most effective demonstration, attention should be paid to the effects of these model characteristics.

Guidance
It is generally believed that tasks will be more effectively learned

if error is minimised in the first stages of learning. Guidance refers to methods by which this is achieved. Subjects are guided through a task in such a way that they are sure to perform the correct movements in the initial stages. Holding (1965) lists four methods of guiding subjects on perceptual and motor tasks: *physical restriction*, whereby a subject is harnessed so that he has to make the correct movements; *forced-response*, whereby he is physically placed into the correct position; *visual guidance*, which involves providing visual cues as an additional source of information; and *verbal guidance*, which is, in effect, giving verbal instructions to a subject on the best way of performing the task. As with other aspects of skills learning, the utility of a particular form of guidance will depend to a large extent on the nature of the task. Physical restriction, for example, will be of little use for tasks that do not involve motor movements. Verbal guidance will be of little help if subjects cannot translate the instructions into practice. A major issue concerns the degree to which subjects should experience errors in order to learn more effectively. When a subject who has experienced guidance in the early stages of learning comes to practise a task without guidance he may find it difficult to adjust to the range of alternative actions that have become available to him. Therefore, some prior experience of unguided trials is generally considered beneficial. Or in the absence of such experience, practice of alternative responses should be built into the learning sequence so that the subject learns to choose the most appropriate action. The nature and extent of guidance in a particular task will be determined by similar considerations to those raised by extrinsic feedback. Thus, if subjects become excessively dependent on the additional information provided by either method, at the expense of the information intrinsic to the task itself, then in the long run their progress will be impaired. Guidance should be used in order to enhance the information in the task, not to replace it.

Summary of experimental findings
Practice, feedback, demonstration and guidance are four variables shown to be important in perceptual and motor skills learning. The general points made about these variables undoubtedly mask the complexity of the subject matter and are, at best, simple generalisations. Thus an effective skills training programme

should involve the demonstration of the skills, or components of it, by a model similar to the subjects but not perceived as an 'expert'. With very complex skills visual guidance may help. Subjects might be guided through the initial stages in order to minimise error, but should be given some practice at alternative responses. Repeated practice is an essential part of the programme. With a complex task practice of components of the task is necessary, but care should be taken that this is compatible with practice of the task as a whole, and the time and effort is not wasted on minor components. It is also best to have brief, frequent sessions, rather than to carry out lengthy, massed trials infrequently, as the former should lead to immediate improvements and maintain motivation. Finally, subjects should receive clear and informative feedback on their performance. This could take place both concurrently during the trial and terminally when the trial is completed. The most useful terminal feedback is that which enhances the feedback intrinsic to the task itself so that subjects can learn to respond successfully when performing without extra feedback. This is particularly important with regard to ensuring successful generalisation.

Description of training

Clinical, educational and industrial training programmes can and do fit into the model derived from the experimental work on perceptual and motor skills. The following is a fairly commonly found programme in all three fields.

There are two important preliminary steps. Firstly, it is necessary to draw up a list of the main problem situations to be faced by those being trained; this can be done by 'critical incident' surveys, or more informally by consulting a number of experienced practitioners – of selling, interviewing, teaching or whatever is being taught. Secondly, it is necessary to find out the best social techniques for dealing with the problem situations. A certain amount of research material is available and this can be supplemented by knowledge of the general principles of social interaction. The whole skill is divided up into a number of smaller units which can be taught separately – sometimes as many as 12–15 in the case of teacher training (see below).

The first phase of each session usually consists of guidance and demonstration. The trainer describes the behaviour to be taught; this involves introducing the trainee to a number of new terms, for example describing the elements of social behaviour, which may require demonstrations by him. The modelling may be given by the trainer, or may be provided by a specially-made videotape, illustrating good and bad performance of the skill in question.

The second phase is practice. A problem situation is defined, and role partners are produced for trainees to practice with, typically for 7–15 minutes. The background of the situation may be filled in with written materials, such as the application form of candidates for interview, or background information about personnel problems; the role partners may be carefully trained beforehand to provide various problems, such as talking too much, or having elaborate and plausible excuses.

The third phase is feedback. There is a feedback session, consisting of verbal comments by the trainer, discussion with other trainees, and playback of audio and video-tapes. Verbal feedback is used to draw attention, constructively and tactfully, to what the trainee was doing wrong, and to suggest alternative styles of behaviour. The tape-recordings provide clear evidence for the accuracy of what is being said. Feedback is found to be more effective when given as soon as possible. Giving feedback is itself a rather difficult social skill. It must be tactful and gentle enough not to upset the trainee, but strong and clear enough to have some impact on his behaviour.

Training can be conducted without the use of any specialised equipment, but it is greatly assisted if certain laboratory arrangements are available. An ideal set-up for interviewer training is shown in figure 4.1. The action takes place on one side of a one-way screen, and is observed by the trainer and other trainees. The use of the microphone is explained below.

There has been a lot of discussion and some research on whether all parts of the programme are necessary. (1) The video-tape recording can be omitted, but most research shows that training is more effective if it is included (Ivey 1971). (2) The trainer can be omitted, and trainees simply compare the video-tape of their performance with the model tapes. This economises on the time of trainers, but a number of experimental studies have shown that microteaching is more effective if there is a trainer to focus attention on details of the playback (Peck and Tucker 1973). (3) The

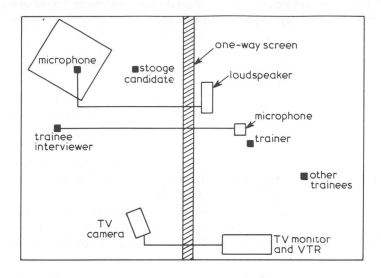

modelling can be omitted, but a variety of studies have shown that training is more effective when it is included.

Skills training requires people to think of everyday behaviour in unfamiliar ways. The use of specialised verbal labels to categorise behaviour can help to bring the elements of the new skill under cognitive control. For example, teachers trained with the categories devised by Flanders (1970) are found to improve their questioning techniques and to concentrate on stimulating self-directed pupil behaviour.

One problem in training is that the trainees have to transfer what they have learned in miniature or in the lab to the real-life situation. The best solution appears to be to hold the training sessions intermittently, to ask the trainees to carry out specific tasks in the real situation, and to report on their progress.

There are several variations on the basic training theme. (1) Role reversal. Here the trainee plays a complementary role to the one he is learning. For example, those who have difficulty with people in authority role-play their own boss. (2) An ear-microphone is inserted in one of the trainee's ears, so that he can be given instructions during the role-playing. This is useful for people who can't think of what to say. (3) More elaborate simulations can be set up, including several persons occupying different roles, environmental props, and so on.

CLINICAL APPLICATIONS

Social skills training

Social skills training as developed by the authors is firmly based on skills theory and the experimental research into social interaction which has been carried out at the Department of Experimental Psychology, Oxford, and in similar laboratories elsewhere (Argyle 1969, 1975). Social skills training has recently become a widely used therapy, particularly in hospitals and out-patient clinics in Britain, Europe and the U.S.A.

Our own method of training (fully described in the manual) follows the social skills model in two respects. Firstly, it uses the basic principles of skills acquisition of guidance, demonstration, practice and feedback as described above. Patients also carry out role-play simulations of situations they find difficult, and better responses are shaped by using knowledge of normal social skill. These tasks are then set as between-session homework assignments. Second, the content of skills training is divided up along the lines suggested in the model, namely perception (or observation) skills, performance skills and cognitive skills. Some of the basic skills described in the manual are:

Getting information Reading social signals	Observation skills
Listening skills Speaking skills Meshing Non-verbal expression Greetings and partings Initiating conversations Rewarding skills Assertive skills	Performance skills
Planning Problem solving	Cognitive skills

There is a growing number of training manuals available, both published and unpublished, some of which are similar to our own; others are quite different in that they do not include perception and cognitive skills or research knowledge of social interaction and non-verbal communication as reviewed in chapter 2. Goldstein (1973) uses a somewhat similar procedure in a treatment package he calls *Structured Learning Therapy*. Patients are seen in groups of 8 to 12, with two therapists. A series of videotapes depicting specific social skills are shown and patients are required to role-play the interaction they have seen. The therapists and other patients provide feedback and encouragement, and homework assignments are given. Goldstein also draws at least partly on a social skills model. For example, he emphasises the need for spaced practice and the provision of appropriate feedback. Another similar training programme called *Personal Effectiveness Training* has been developed by Liberman *et al.* (1975).

The majority of social skills training programmes have been carried out using videotapes either as feedback or to demonstrate interactions. This is quite an expensive form of therapy both in terms of personnel and equipment (though not in time). Marzillier, Lambert and Kellett (1976) developed a more economical method, whereby interactions were modelled by the therapist and feedback was provided by the therapist's comments and audiotaped recordings. At a later stage role-playing was extended to encompass interaction with people other than the therapist. Some training methods have been criticised for not including transfer training to aid the generalisation of skills to outside situations. Falloon *et al.* (1974) are among those who have devised an 'Operant Home Programme' which includes specified homework tasks, a self-reinforcement scheme, accountability to a named friend or relative, and all-patient meetings between sessions.

Other training packages have used cognitive-based methods on the one hand (Christensen *et al.* 1974) and sensitivity training methods on the other (Johnson 1972).

Some training programmes have specialised in skills at certain levels. (i) Perception skills: Davitz (1964) developed a method for improving perception of other people's emotions from tones of voice. During training, groups of 3–8 subjects listened to a practice tape in which letters of the alphabet were read with different emotional expressions, and they tried to identify the emotions; during a second playing they were told which emotions were to be expressed before each item; they later tried to express the emotions themselves, and their attempts were discussed by the group. The training occupied several 15-minute sessions. An excellent example of an alternative training procedure is given by an experiment in which interpretations of bodily movements were made more accurate. Jecker *et al.* (1965) succeeded in training teachers to perceive more accurately whether or not pupils had understood what they were being taught. The measure consisted of a series of one-minute films showing children being taught; a subsequent question to the child (not shown on the film) found out if he really had understood. By showing teachers these films, and by drawing attention to the behavioural and facial cues for comprehension, it was possible to increase their scores on a new set of similar films. Another method is to instruct trainees in rating various aspects of interaction, and to give them practice at recording the behaviour of other trainees. They can learn to record such things as number and length of speeches, an elementary categorisation of social acts, duration of eye-contact or direction of gaze at each other, number of speech errors and so on.

(ii) Problem-solving skills. Spivack and Shure (1974) trained disturbed children and adolescents in cognitive skills to solve interpersonal problems, imagine alternative responses and evaluate their consequences. This consisted of a series of games in which the concepts of decision-making were learned. For instance, they were taught the use of the word '*or*' in considering alternative responses (e.g. 'You could do A *or* you could do B'), the words '*if . . . then*' and '*because*' in evaluating consequences, the word '*and*' in considering more than one attribute about a person or situation, the word '*might*' or '*maybe*' for considering ambiguity in situations. Spivack and Shure report considerable success in reducing aggressive behaviour and increasing awareness of others' preferences and feelings. They report significant differences between normal and hospitalised psychiatric adults and adolescents, and are developing training programmes for these groups.

Assertive training
Assertive training is one of the oldest behavioural methods of treatment. It was developed by Joseph Wolpe (1958) as a treatment for neurotic disorders, drawing on the ideas and practice of Andrew Salter (1949). Wolpe uses this technique – often in conjunction with another behavioural technique, systematic

desensitisation – for those patients who are excessively passive and submissive in their social and work relationships. Wolpe's technique consists fundamentally of breaking down the problem into specific components and advising his patients on how to be more assertive. If necessary, Wolpe instigates 'behaviour rehearsal', i.e. role-playing of the interaction on several occasions to give the patient practice in assertive responses. At times Wolpe demonstrates the appropriate assertive behaviour by means of 'role-reversal', namely by adopting the patient's role in the interaction, while the patient takes the alternative role. Finally, Wolpe suggests tasks for the patient to carry out outside therapy. These are graded in terms of difficulty in the hope that the patient's initial attempts at assertiveness will meet with success. At subsequent sessions, the patient reports on his progress or his difficulties (Wolpe 1958, 1970, 1973b).

The salient features of Wolpe's procedures are thus modelling, advice, role-playing, task-assignment and the reinforcement of assertive behaviour. The treatment generally takes place on an individual basis within the therapist's office without the use of other personnel or any special equipment. The original meaning of 'assertiveness' was that of 'standing up for one's rights', and Wolpe's technique has always emphasised this particular aspect of social interaction (Wolpe 1958). However, he now defines the term more broadly as '. . . the proper expression of any emotion other than anxiety towards another person' (Wolpe 1973a). Among a list of assertive statements he makes a distinction between *hostile* and *commendatory* statements, the latter consisting of paying compliments and direct expressions of positive feelings. Wolpe theorises that assertive training serves to de-condition neurotic anxiety. It provides the opportunity for alternative responses to take the place of maladaptive anxiety-based behaviour.

A number of variations of the treatment method have been introduced. In particular, videotape recordings have been employed to emphasise non-verbal components of assertiveness (Eisler, Miller and Hersen 1973) and audiotape recordings have been used as additional feedback (McFall and Marston 1970). Patients have been treated in small groups as well as individually (e.g. Bloomfield 1973). These developments have served to enhance the modelling component of the therapy, by extending the range of interactions that can be portrayed. Moreover, the recordings can be used to focus on particular components of assertive skills. There has also been some attempt to break down assertiveness into its verbal and non-verbal components but relatively few studies have explored this important feature of the training in any depth.

A typical assertive training session may proceed as follows: (i) the therapist describes a problem situation; (ii) the subject responds out loud into a tape recorder; (iii) the subject listens to the tape-recorded responses of a male and then a female model; (iv) the therapist guides the subject regarding what makes a good assertive response in the situation; (v) the subject hears or watches a replay of his response and reflects on it; (vi) the subject responds again. The following example is taken from McFall and Lillesand (1971) and was used for unassertive students.

> *Therapist*: A person in your class, whom you do not know very well, borrowed your notes weeks ago, then failed to return them, thus forcing you to take notes on scrap paper. Now this person comes up to you again and says, 'Hey, mind if I borrow your class notes again?' What do you say? (Subject practises responding.) Now listen to the response of two assertive subjects to this same situation.
>
> *Male model*: 'You didn't return my notes last time, so I'm not going to lend them to you this time.'
>
> *Female model*: 'No, I just can't be sure you're going to have them back in time.'
>
> *Therapist* (coaching): Notice that both these assertive subjects let the person know that their refusal was based on his past behaviour. Their responses were brief and without any ambiguity. Their voices expressed some irritation over the past behaviour of this person, but in general their responses were well controlled. Now listen to your response to this situation and compare it to the responses of the models you have just heard. (Playback) Now you will hear the same situation again. This time try to make your responses more assertive. (Repeat situation; subject practises responding.)

The main difference between assertive training and social skills training is the broader based nature of the latter approach. Whereas assertive training aims to deal specifically with lack of assertiveness, defined as excessive submissiveness and an inability to express positive emotions, social skills training aims to deal with any deficits in social performance whether characterised as lack of assertiveness or other social difficulty. Social skills training, for example, is often used to teach patients simply to say more when interacting with others, or to reward the other person by attending closely, smiling, etc. There are other differences; for instance, social skills training emphasises non-verbal behaviour more, and the use of videotape feedback. Nevertheless, there is also considerable overlap between them as they are currently practised and, to a certain extent, the distinction between them is a result of historical accident.

PROFESSIONAL AND OTHER APPLICATIONS

The full training package of guidance, demonstration, practice and feedback has, in recent years, become a rather more developed and standard training procedure in professional than in clinical settings. This form of training is now used in most colleges for teachers, for training interviewers and counsellors and for industrial social skills training. Since the procedure is so similar, experience in these fields can be of value to psychiatric applications, and vice versa.

Microteaching

This is now the most widely used form of training, and is becoming very common in the U.S.A. and Britain. The trainer explains some aspect of teaching skills, e.g. asking questions, and shows a video-tape or film of a good teacher doing it well. A trainee then teaches a prepared lesson, lasting 5, 10 or 25 minutes. The class consists of five to six children (her own, in the case of in-service teaching. There are at least as many sessions as there are components to be taught (Peck and Tucker 1973).

The most commonly taught component skills of teaching are:

1. structuring, induction of set
2. reinforcement, verbal and non-verbal
3. asking questions, including higher-order, divergent and probing questions
4. lecturing, explaining
5. illustration, use of examples
6. encouraging pupil participation
7. stimulus variation, enthusiasm

8. closure of lesson
9. elimination of bad habits.

After the lesson, the videotape is played back and commented on by the trainer. The lesson is then repeated and the second videotape played back.

Counselling

Similar training methods have been developed to teach the counselling skills recommended by Carkhuff (1969). The procedure is as follows:

1. The trainee receives instruction to enter a room where he will interview a client. Depending on the situation, the topic may or may not be defined. Similar instructions are given to the volunteer client, with the exception that he is told he is about to be interviewed.

2. A five-minute diagnostic session (with the trainee interviewing the client) is then videotaped.

3. The client leaves the room and completes an evaluation form; or may be interviewed by a second supervisor. These data are then available for the supervisory session with the trainee.

4. The trainee reads a written manual describing the specific skill to be learned in this session. The supervisor talks with him about the session and the manual.

5. Video models of an expert demonstrating the specific skill are shown. There may be a positive and negative model of the skill.

6. The trainee is shown his initial interview and discusses this with his supervisor. He is asked to identify examples where he practised, or failed to apply, the specific skill in question.

7. The supervisor and trainee review the skill together and plan for the next counselling session.

8. The trainee reinterviews the same client for five minutes.

9. Feedback and evaluation on the final session are made available to the trainee.

The specific skills which are taught are as follows:

1. *Beginning skills*
   (a) Attending behaviour
   (b) Open invitation to talk
   (c) Minimal encouragement to talk

2. *Listening skills : selective attention*
   (a) Reflection and summary of feeling
   (b) Paraphrasing
3. *Skills of self-expression*
   (a) Expression of feeling
   (b) Expression of content
   (c) Direct mutual communication
4. *Interpretation (Ivey 1971)*   (Ivey 1971)

Interviewing

A system for training selection interviewing was devised by
Sidney and Argyle (1969). Two sets of problem situations are used.
The first set consists of the most common kinds of awkward
candidate:

talks too much

talks too little

asks too many questions

very nervous

over self-presentation

class or cultural difference

unrewarding

female behaves amorously

not very interested in job

neurotic

Trainees conduct short interviews with trained confederates who
act these parts; amateur actors have been found to be the most
successful in these roles. If the trainee is quite unable to cope with
a confederate, the interview is interrupted and he is given further
instructions.

The second set consists of asking trainees to assess, one at
a time, a number of the most relevant personality traits – intelligence, judgment, creativity, authoritarianism, neuroticism,
self-image, social competence, and achievement motivation. After
each interview a discussion is held about what rating (on a 7-point
scale) the 'candidate' should be given in the trait in question.
When a complete profile has been obtained for a candidate, a
discussion is held on his overall suitability for various kinds of job.

Learning on the job

This is probably the most common way in which people learn social skills. They learn by sheer practice, or they are helped by a trainer or supervisor who may give verbal guidance or intervene in other ways. Learning on the job has an inherent advantage over other forms of training in that there is no problem of transferring newly-learned skills from the training lab to the real situation.

However, there is plenty of evidence that learning on the job often fails to take place. Learning social skills simply by doing them can be remarkably unsuccessful. Fiedler (1970) found that the more years of experience industrial supervisors had the *less* effective they were. Argyle *et al.* (1958) found that supervisors often learned the *wrong* things by experience, e.g. to use close, punitive and authoritarian styles of supervision. Quite simple aspects of social skills may not be learned – for example, some very experienced interviewers are unable to deal with candidates who won't talk. Further, perceptual discrimination may fail to improve; Jecker *et al.* (1965) found that experienced teachers were no better than beginners at judging whether children had understood or not.

The reasons why learning on the job often fails to work are easy to understand, if one considers the four probable processes involved in learning.

(i) Trainees find out by trial and error which social techniques are most effective. Trial and error may fail because there is often no clear or immediate feedback on the success of some style of behaviour. For example, research on teaching shows that pupil achievement is greater when teachers use positive reinforcement, make use of pupils' ideas, ask higher-order questions, structure lessons, are businesslike, well-organised and enthusiastic, use a variety of methods and materials, are clear, audible and easy to understand, and do not make much use of criticism (Rosenshine 1971). There would be no way of discovering these effects short of doing systematic research. In addition, trainees might never hit on the best social techniques by trial and error. To make silent interview candidates talk it is necessary to use open-ended questions and to give systematic reinforcement when the candidate replies; this style might never be discovered without instruction. When clear feedback is given it is very effective. Gage *et al.* (1960) asked 3900 school children to fill in rating scales to describe their ideal teacher and how their actual teachers behaved; the results were shown to half of the teachers, who subsequently improved on ten of the twelve scales, compared with the no-feedback group. In most situations this kind of feedback is not available.

(ii) Trainees imitate the social skills of successful performers. Imitation of others may fail because immediate superiors often do not use the best social skills themselves, and in any case it may be difficult to know which aspects of their behaviour should be imitated and which not.

(iii) Trainees occupy reciprocal roles in relation to others, and will adopt behaviour appropriate to their role in response to others' behaviour. Acquisition of appropriate role behaviour may be impeded if there is some degree of role-conflict. Children may elicit certain patterns of response from teachers, for example, but these will not necessarily be the most effective styles of teaching.

(iv) Trainees are instructed and coached by supervisors. Coaching may fail to take place, because the trainer is too busy or is not a good instructor. Ideally he should be an expert on the job, be sensitised to the elements and sequences of behaviour involved, and be able to talk about them. He should observe the trainee in action regularly and hold coaching and feedback sessions.

Examples of learning on the job.   Sales.   There is usually very little training apart from what is learned on the job. A study by Argyle and colleagues of newly-appointed salesgirls in a department store showed that their volume of sales rose steadily over the first eight months and then levelled off – at 90 per cent over the starting level where there was an individual bonus, and about 50 per cent where there was a group bonus or no bonus (Argyle 1972). However, some girls did not improve at all, while others got worse.

Psychotherapy.   This is usually taught on the job, the trainee either being present, watching over closed-circuit television, or examining the notes taken. In the Truax and Carkhuff (1967) system of training, use is made of tape-recordings to present models, trainee therapists are taught the use of rating scales, and emphasis is placed throughout on empathy, warmth and genuineness. The training takes at least one hundred hours.

Teaching.   Apart from the use of micro-teaching, trainee teachers are usually placed under the direction of an experienced teacher, who may or may not function as an efficient instructor of social skills. Another approach is to train teachers, on the job, in the use of special reinforcement procedures. For example, teachers can be taught to reinforce appropriate behaviour and to punish by ignoring deviant behaviour, by themselves being reinforced. The teacher is trained by the trainer reinforcing the teacher for reinforcing the child correctly!

Educational methods

It may be possible to teach social skills by more traditional teaching methods. It is important to explore these methods since they are much cheaper and more widely available than those described so far – which need specially qualified trainers or expensive equipment. *Lectures*, followed by discussion, can be given in which various aspects of skill are explained. They may focus on the basic principles of social behaviour, or on the details of recommended social techniques. The lectures may be followed by discussion among the trainees, or there may be guided discussion without lectures. Follow-up studies show that lectures on human relations lead to improved scores on questionnaires, but it has not been shown that any behavioural changes in skill are produced. There are certain difficulties about lectures. They are no good unless the audience is really interested in what the lecturer has to say, or unless he can make them interested by the forcefulness of his presentation, and has a manner and status which make him personally acceptable.

Another group method is the discussion of *case studies*, as is often done in management training. These consist of problem situations to which the group has to find the best solution; they may be presented as filmstrips or in written form. Case studies are used for general education in management problems, but can also be focussed entirely on the human relations aspects. The main weakness is that trainees do not acquire any general principles, though there can be increased awareness of the human relations aspects of problems. It might be possible to devise case studies in such a way that they would illustrate and draw attention to basic principles; perhaps if a large enough number of cases were used, trainees could be helped to make inductive generalisations from them.

This method has recently been used for teaching social skills to school children. A case is presented by the teacher, or from a text book, which illustrates problems such as dealing with authority, emotional problems at home, or moral dilemmas. The case is then discussed by the class under the guidance of the teacher (McPhail 1972). Similar methods are used in the teaching of psychiatrists.

Reading is one of the traditional methods of learning, but can social skills be learned in this way? There are a number of books in this area, such as *How to Win Friends and Influence People* (Carnegie 1936), but there is no evidence as to the influence they have.

We have already referred to the use of *films* in connection with role-playing. A number of training films are now available for social skills training, such as those made by Sidney and Argyle (1969). However, no follow-up studies are yet available on the use of films for this purpose. Films have been used for training in *manual* skills for some time, and these are found to be successful under certain conditions – if the learner has to try out part of the skill after each piece of film, if the film is shot from his point of view, e.g. over his shoulder, and if appropriate use is made of slow motion, animation and sequences of stills, showing the successive steps in the skill. Again, it looks as if films can play an important part in an overall training scheme, but are not much good alone.

Dynamic techniques

Psychotherapy and allied techniques are an alternative approach to skills training, in that they often have similar objectives but, as we shall see, use entirely different methods, for they aim to bring about psychological or 'dynamic' change within an individual which should then lead to changes in his behaviour.

SENSITIVITY TRAINING

Although this method is labelled 'training', it differs radically from the other training methods discussed so far, in that the process is not didactic but experimental; that is, clients are intended to benefit from participation in such groups not because they are taught particular skills but as a result of their immediate and direct experiences within the groups (Rogers 1975). So, although the goals of sensitivity training include improved social skills and effectiveness in social situations, more emphasis is placed on sensitivity to others and interpersonal phenomena, as well as improved self-understanding and self-acceptance.

The style and format of such groups can vary considerably, ranging from T-groups, where the interaction is primarily verbal, to sensitivity groups proper with various exercises to encourage intimacy, to other kinds of groups involving catharsis by screaming and aggression with the use of padded clubs. There is no fixed or accepted method of conducting a sensitivity group, and it seems that the personality and personal philosophy of the group leader will largely determine the way a group develops (Lieberman, Yalom and Miles 1973). Group sessions can be conducted on a regular weekly basis, or for several hours at a time, or for as long as a whole weekend as in the Marathon Group encounters, again depending on the views of the leader and also of the group members themselves.

Some of the training techniques used can be mentioned briefly.

(i) *T-groups*

The trainer takes a backseat and leaves the group to decide how to run itself; discussion of what happens in the group is then the focus of attention. For example, there may be a struggle for dominance, members have to decide whom they like and don't like, there may be a male-female pairing, and some people may fail to participate. The trainer shows the group how to express their feelings and reactions to one another, he encourages openness, and provides a model of participatory leadership. There may be other kinds of training as well, such as role-playing, lectures and discussion (Bradford, Gibb and Benne 1964).

(ii) *Encounter groups*

There is no standard procedure, though sets of exercises have been described by Schutz and others. For example, individuals who have difficulty in giving and receiving affection may be put through the following routines:

> 'Give and take affection'. One person stands in the centre of a circle with his eyes shut; the others approach him and express their feelings towards him non-verbally in whatever way they choose – usually by hugging, stroking, massaging, lifting, etc.

'Roll and rock'. One person stands in the centre of the circle, relaxed and with his eyes shut; the group pass him round from person to person, taking his weight. The group then pick him up and sway him gently backwards and forwards, very quietly. (Schutz 1967).

In less bodily-oriented groups 'immediate intimacy' exercises are used, in which members pair off and spend one minute telling one another the most important things about themselves, then two things they are proud of, and then two things they are ashamed of. Another exercise sometimes used is role-reversal, where, for example, pairs of members try to adopt each other's style of behaviour.

The effects of sensitivity training are that about one-third benefit while 10 per cent are worse (e.g. Lieberman *et al.* 1973).

One lesson to be drawn is that we should be careful that forms of training do not distress trainees or patients unduly. Psychiatrically disturbed individuals are particularly at risk, and it may be that as a rule they should not be placed in such groups.

PSYCHODRAMA

Although traditionally associated with the dynamic techniques, psychodrama owes them no theoretical allegiance, being similar only in its emphasis on 'spontaneity' or 'creativity' – the creed of its founder J. L. Moreno (1946). It can be used equally in the pursuit of catharsis, insight, modelling, desensitisation, social skills and assertive training, and so on. It therefore provides a potential bridge between the analytic, interactional and behavioural models of treatment (Kennard 1976).

Psychodrama differs from conventional group therapy in that a problem belonging to one member of the group is given concrete shape by the enactment in the group of an actual or potential situation exemplifying the problem.

There are three stages. The first of these is the 'warm-up', in which free discusson or various exercises take place – depending on the style of the therapist. Following this, the leader selects a 'protagonist' and encourages him to talk about the problem he has raised and about particular situations associated with it which he can recall or imagine. To aid him, the leader, or 'director', may suggest that he and the protagonist walk round the room while they talk. This is a step towards getting 'into' the action. The director then selects from the situations mentioned by the protagonist one that may serve as a useful starting point. This may be related to the immediate problem – e.g. a row at home, frustration at work, indecision over a particular issue, anxiety about a forthcoming event – or may be related to an earlier episode which contained the seeds of the present problem.

At this point the director will use one or more of a number of techniques. One is the empty chair technique, where the protagonist is asked to picture a significant other person in the chair and talk to him in the way he would like to. Another is to ask the protagonist to choose someone to play this person – to be an 'antagonist' – and to 'role in' the chosen member by giving him information about the attitudes and feelings (as seen by the protagonist) of this person. A third technique is that of 'role-reversal', where the protagonist and antagonist change places. At this stage, other members of the group may be asked to 'double' for one or other of those engaged in the action. They do this by standing closely behind one of the chairs, placing their hands on the shoulders of the person in the chair, and speaking as if they were that person.

Further elaboration may take place with other antagonists, the reconstruction of different scenes, the switch to imaginary or potential conversations and so on. At all times the director, who may work with a co-director, maintains control over the choice of scenes, the level of emotional impact which they may have, and the general direction of the proceedings. He has the choice of whether to help the protagonist explore one particular relationship, or certain types of situations, or to try alternative ways of behaving.

A final, and important, stage is the feedback. Here, the antagonists are 'de-roled', revealing how it felt to be the person that the protagonist made them. The rest of the group are invited to share aspects of their own experience.

Psychodrama aims to help people share their problems; to clarify the emotional components in a situation, expecially those which affect interpersonal perception; to help the protagonist see what he looks like from the chair of his adversary, and to hear the 'doubles' of the rest of the group. It also aims to improve empathy in the group, and to 'defuse' the anxiety or fear of an awaited meeting or other situation.

So far there have been few attempts to study the effects of psychodrama experimentally, but the technique is an interesting one which can be of direct use in social skills training.

PSYCHOTHERAPY

Psychotherapy is the treatment of interpersonal problems by means of conversation of a special kind between therapist and patient. The conversation can take a variety of forms, the most influential probably being Freudian psychoanalysis and its subsequent developments, Jungian analytical psychology and Rogerian non-directive therapy. However, all forms of psychotherapy are similar in creating a strong interpersonal bond, in encouraging the patient to talk about his troubles, in trying to understand his thoughts and feelings, in giving him insight into his problems by interpreting these and encouraging him to take active steps to solve them. Improvement in social behaviour can be brought about indirectly by insight and the resolution of inner conflict.

Because of the different schools of thought in psychotherapy, one cannot generalise about the approach to social inadequacy. However, most psychotherapists, especially those with a psychoanalytic orientation, look at social inadequacy in a quite different way from social skills therapists. Their approach may consist of interpretation of the motivations responsible for the inadequacy; for instance, if the individual can't make friends it may be because he has a deep-rooted fear of intimate relationships. Social skills therapists, on the other hand, suppose that what is lacking is social skill, due to a failure in one or more of its various components. More research is needed to reconcile these points of view. Undoubtedly there is scope for a joint approach.

There are schools of psychotherapy which maintain that social inadequacy plays a central part in neurosis, notably Sullivan, Fairbairn and Berne (see Argyle 1969). However, the therapy practised still consists of conversation between therapist and patient. Some psychotherapists have regarded the interaction between therapist and patient as a form of training in social behaviour which may generalise to other relationships. However, this is social behaviour of a very special kind, and it seems unlikely that it would afford very useful practice. In group therapy, on the other hand, there is opportunity to establish relationships with a wider variety of people.

Some therapists emphasise cognitive processes. For example, Ellis (1957) found that neurotics often hold certain mistaken ideas, some of them in the interpersonal sphere; for example, 'it is necessary to be loved and approved by everyone', or 'certain people are bad and should be punished'. In this method of rational psychotherapy, Ellis gets the patient to take action that will show him that these assumptions are wrong, shows the patient how they are causing his distress, and teaches him to rethink them. This has something in common with aspects of social skills training, such as explanation of the dynamics of situations.

Studies of psychotherapy show improvement for about 66 per cent and deterioration for about 10 per cent. There is a great deal of controversy over whether the improved patients would have recovered spontaneously anyway, and this is still an open question. Middle-class, less disturbed, younger, intelligent and well motivated patients seem to do better, and therapists who are high on 'empathy, warmth and genuineness', and similar in background to the patient, are more effective.

Milieu treatment

Milieu treatment refers to a planned therapeutic environment in a mental hospital or other residential unit. We shall consider briefly two main kinds of milieu – therapeutic communities and token economies.

THERAPEUTIC COMMUNITIES

Therapeutic communities were designed by Maxwell Jones (1952) and others to avoid the 'institutionalising' effects of ordinary mental hospitals in which patients may become completely dependent on the hospital and lose touch with the outside world. They planned, in addition, to give patients some preparation for life outside by providing them with regular work and giving them some other responsibility. The usual ingredients are a sheltered workshop, daily meetings at which reports are made about the last twenty-four hours and community decisions are taken, and nurses and doctors out of uniform who adopt a similar status to the patients. Expeditions are encouraged, and the hospital is frequently open to visitors.

There is a certain amount of non-experimental evidence that therapeutic communities, alone or in combination, are able to modify social behaviour. It is not clear how the improved social behaviour is learned – perhaps through imitation of staff and fitting into a set of co-operative social roles. The treatment is to a large extent aimed at modifying social behaviour, with the emphasis on group work, group decisions, and feedback about unsatisfactory social behaviour. It is not, perhaps, the niceties of social skills which are taught so much as a generally increased level of co-operative and sociable behaviour. The benefits are not restricted to educated middle-class neurotic patients, as in the case of psychotherapy.

Therapeutic communities do not lend themselves easily to controlled experimental study, and to date few efforts have been made to validate the technique in this way.

TOKEN ECONOMIES

Therapeutic milieus of the kind just described practise a certain amount of deliberate reinforcement of desired forms of behaviour. In token economies, systematic reinforcement schedules are introduced. Tokens, for example in the form of poker chips, are given when desired behaviour is produced, and the tokens can later be exchanged for food or other desired objects, privileges, and entertainments. The behaviour being trained often includes social behaviour such as being co-operative. Ayllon and Azrin (1968) established a token community in a schizophrenic ward and found that many aspects of patient behaviour improved greatly, but it is not reported whether there were any long-term effects. The effects of token communities in improving behaviour on the ward have been reported in a number of studies, though many of these suffer from methodological and design problems which make results hard to interpret. In one of the best controlled studies to date, Baker and Hall (1975) found that the token system left schizophrenic symptomatology largely unaffected but was able to promote the skills and interests which enable patients to cope with their illness and to live fuller lives.

Symptom treatments

Some treatments are aimed at eradicating or suppressing symptoms directly, and the two main forms now in general use are behaviour therapy and drugs. The symptoms most successfully alleviated are anxiety and obsessionality in the neuroses, and florid behaviour and mood swings in the psychoses. All of these are known to disrupt social behaviour, and their alleviation can often restore normal functioning in non-psychotic conditions if there is no underlying social inadequacy. Where symptoms and social inadequacy are both present, an approach combining both training and symptom treatment can and has been successfully used (e.g. Hallam 1974).

BEHAVIOUR THERAPY

Behaviour therapy has been most successfully used in eradicating 'fears and phobias' (Marks 1969), and more recently obsessionality (Rachman *et al.*, 1973; Hackmann and McLean 1975). The best known and most widely used form is systematic desensitisation (Wolpe 1958), in which the patient is asked to imagine or take part in an anxiety-provoking situation while in a state of deep relaxation. The patient works his way up a hierarchy of self-selected situations, graded according to difficulty. Each situation is presented on several occasions until it fails to elicit further anxiety. Wolpe's theory is that the technique works by a process of counter-conditioning – the relaxation counters and thus diminishes or eradicates the anxiety. Though the theory has not stood up well to experimental studies, the practice has (Yates 1975).

An increasingly used anxiety-reduction technique is 'flooding' (Stampfl and Levis 1967), which consists of prolonged exposure, in imagination or practice, to situations that provoke maximum anxiety, until that anxiety is diminished.

Modelling is an anxiety-reduction technique (Bandura 1969) producing similar results to the above two therapies, but works mainly by exposure to a model who participates in progressively more fear-provoking activities.

Recently, a number of modifications have been made which increase the effectiveness of some of these therapies. For instance, in 'covert modelling' the fearful subject can simply *imagine* a model engaging in various activities (Cautela 1971). Another development combines aspects of desensitisation and modelling in a technique called 'guided participation' (Bandura *et al.* 1969).

Most of these techniques, which are only a small sample of those in use or actively under development, work more effectively by getting the patient to change his 'self-instructions', i.e. by telling himself he will cope rather than that he will fail (Meichenbaum 1974).

Some of them have also been used experimentally in assertive and social skills training, and these developments will be discussed in chapter 5.

DRUGS

Drugs are widely used in psychiatric treatment, often in combination with other forms of treatment. The main drugs are the minor tranquillizers for neurosis, chlorpromazine for schizophrenia, and the anti-depressants. There is a tendency to make more use of drugs, and less use of psychotherapy, with working-class patients.

How can drugs improve social behaviour? Generally they are used in combination with other forms of treatment. By relaxing the patient, and, at least temporarily, removing excessive anxiety, drugs make it possible to treat otherwise inaccessible patients by other means. However, drugs can lead to improvements, at any rate on a temporary basis, without other treatment, especially for psychotics. We must suppose that the removal of, for example, excessive anxiety or depression, enables the patient to use what basic social skills he possesses.

Conclusion

The techniques described in this chapter cover a wide spectrum, and the question arises: which ones work best? There is an extensive literature on most of these techniques and it would be impossible to attempt an overall evaluation in this book. Instead, we shall confine ourselves in the next chapter to a critical evaluation of skills training and allied methods.

References

ANNETT, J. (1969) *Feedback and Human Behaviour*. Harmondsworth: Penguin.
ARGYLE, M. (1969) *Social Interaction*. London: Methuen.

ARGYLE, M. (1972) *The Psychology of Interpersonal Behaviour*, 2nd edition. Harmondsworth: Penguin.

ARGYLE, M. (1975) *Bodily Communication*. London: Methuen.

ARGYLE, M., GARDNER, G. AND CIOFFI, F. (1958) Supervisory methods related to productivity, absenteeism and labour turnover. *Human Relations*, 11, 23–45.

AYLLON, T. AND AZRIN, N. H. (1968) *The Token Economy : a Motivational System for Therapy and Rehabilitation*. New York: Appleton-Century-Crofts.

BAKER, R. AND HALL, J. (1975) A controlled study of a Token Economy. Paper prepared for the Annual Conference of the British Association for Behavioural Psychotherapy, York, 1975.

BANDURA, A. (1969) *Principles of Behavior Modification*. New York: Holt, Rinehart and Winston.

BANDURA, A. (1971) *Social Learning Theory*. Morristown, New Jersey: General Learning Press.

BANDURA, A., BLANCHARD, E. B. AND RITTER, S. (1969) Relative efficacy of desensitization and modeling approaches for inducing behavioral affective and attitudinal changes. *Journal of Personality and Social Psychology*, 13, 173–200.

BARLOW, D. H. AND HERSEN, M. (1973) Single-case experimental designs. Uses in applied research. *Archives of General Psychiatry*, 29, 319–25.

BILODEAU, E. A. AND BILODEAU, I. MCD. (1958) Variation of temporal intervals among critical events in five studies of knowledge of results. *Journal of Experimental Psychology*, 55, 603–12.

BLOOMFIELD, H. H. (1973) Assertive training in an outpatient group of chronic schizophrenics: a preliminary report. *Behavior Therapy*, 4, 277–81.

BRADFORD, L. P., GIBB, J. R. AND BENNE, K. D. (1964) *T-Group Theory and Laboratory Method*. New York: Wiley.

CARKHUFF, R. R. (1969) *Helping and Human Relations; a Primer for Lay and Professional Helpers*, Vols. I and II. New York: Holt, Rinehart and Winston.

CARNEGIE, D. (1936) *How to Win Friends and Influence People*. New York: Simon and Schuster.

CAUTELA, J. R. (1971) Covert modeling. Paper presented at Fifth Annual Meeting of the Association for Advancement of Behavior Therapy. Washington, D.C.

CHRISTENSEN, C. M., BLOCH, B., BRIEDIS, I., ERSIE, R., HEATH, J. AND SHANNON, H. (1974) 'Development and field testing of an interpersonal coping skills program.' Roneod. Department of Applied Psychology, The Ontario Institute for Studies in Education Research and Development.

CROSSMAN, E. R. F. (1959) A theory of the acquisition of speed skill. *Ergonomics*, 2, 153–66.

DAVITZ, J. R. (1964) *The Communication of Emotional Meaning*. New York: McGraw-Hill.

EISLER, R. M., MILLER, P. M. AND HERSEN, M. (1973) Components of assertive behavior. *Journal of Clinical Psychology*, 29, 295–9.

ELLIS, A. (1957) Rational psychotherapy and individual psychology. *Journal of Individual Psychology*, 13, 38–44.

FALLOON, I., LINDLEY, P. AND MCDONALD, R. (1974) 'Social training: A Manual.' Unpublished manuscript, Maudsley Hospital, London, S.E.5.

FIEDLER, F. E. (1970) Leadership experience and leader effectiveness – another hypothesis shot to hell. *Organisational Behaviour and Human Performance*, 5, 1–14.

FITTS, P. M. AND POSNER, M. I. (1967) *Human Performance*. Monterey, S. Calif.: Brooks/Cole.

FLANDERS, N. A. (1970) *Analysing Teaching Behavior*. Reading, Mass.: Addison-Wesley.

GAGE, N. L., RUNKEL, P. J. AND CHATTERJEE, B. B. (1960) *Equilibrium Theory and Behavior Change: An Experiment in Feedback from Pupils to Teachers*. Urbana, Illinois: Bureau of Educational Research.

GOLDSTEIN, A. P. (1973) *Structured Learning Therapy: Toward a Psychotherapy for the Poor*. New York and London: Academic Press.

GOLDSTEIN, M. AND RITTENHOUSE, C. H. (1954) Knowledge of results in the acquisition and transfer of a gunnery skill. *Journal of Experimental Psychology*, 48, 187–96.

HACKMANN, A. AND MCLEAN, C. (1975) A comparison of flooding, and thought stopping in the treatment of obsessional neurosis. *Behaviour Research and Therapy*, 13, 263–71.

HALLAM, R. S. (1974) Extinction of ruminations: A case study. *Behavior Therapy*, 5, 565–8.

HOLDING, D. H. (1965) *Principles of Training*. Oxford: Pergamon.

IVEY, A. E. (1971) *Microcounseling*. New York: C. C. Thomas.

JECKER, J. D., MACCOBY, N. AND BREITROSE, H. S. (1965) Improving accuracy in interpreting non-verbal cues of comprehension. *Psychology in the Schools*, 2, 239–44.

JOHNSON, D. W. (1972) *Reaching Out: Interpersonal Effectiveness and Self-Actualisation*. Englewood Cliffs, N.J.: Prentice-Hall.

JONES, M. (1952) *Social Psychiatry*. London: Tavistock.

KENNARD, D. (1976) Psychodrama: Theory and Techniques. Lecture given at London Centre for Psychotherapy, October.

KRASNER, L. (1971) The operant approach in behavior therapy. In A. E. Bergin and S. Garfield (eds) *Handbook of Psychotherapy and Behavior Change: an Empirical Analysis*. New York: Wiley.

LEGGE, D. (ed.) (1970) *Skills*. Harmondsworth: Penguin.

LIBERMAN, R. P., KING, L. W., DE RISI, W. AND MCCANN, M. (1975) *Personal Effectiveness*. Champaign, Ill.: Research Press.

LIEBERMAN, M. A., YALOM, I. D. AND MILES, M. B. (1973) *Encounter Groups: First Facts*. New York: Basic Books.

MCFALL, R. M. AND LILLESAND, D. (1971) Behavior rehearsal with modeling and coaching in assertive training. *Journal of Abnormal Psychology*, 77, 313–23

MCFALL, R. M. AND MARSTON, A. R. (1970) An experimental investigation of behavior rehearsal in assertive training. *Journal of Abnormal Psychology*, 76, 295–303.

MCPHAIL, P. (1972) *Moral Education in Secondary Schools*. London: Longmans.

MARKS, I. M. (1969) *Fears and Phobias*. London: Heinemann.

MARZILLIER, J. S., LAMBERT, C. AND KELLETT, J. (1976) A controlled evaluation of systematic desensitization and social skills training for socially inadequate psychiatric patients. *Behavior Research and Therapy*, 14, 225–38.

MEICHENBAUM, D. H. (1971) Examination of model characteristics in reducing avoidance behavior. *Journal of Personality and Social Psychology*, 17, 298–307.

MEICHENBAUM, D. H. (1974) Self-instructional methods. In F. H. Kanfer and A. P. Goldstein (eds) *Helping People Change*. Oxford: Pergamon.

MORENO, J. L. (1946) *Psychodrama*, Vol. 1. New York: Beacon House.

PECK, R. F. AND TUCKER, J. A. (1973) Research on teacher education. In R. M. V. Travers (ed.) *Second Handbook of Research on Teaching*. Chicago, Ill.: Rand McNally.

RACHMAN, S., MARKS, I. M. AND HODGSON, R. (1973) The treatment of obsessive-compulsive neurosis by modelling and flooding in vivo. *Behaviour Research and Therapy*, 11, 463–71.

ROGERS, C. R. (1975) *Encounter Groups*. Harmondsworth: Pelican.

ROSENSHINE, B. (1971) Teaching Behaviour and Student Achievement. Slough: N.F.E.R.

SALTER, A. (1949) *Conditioned Reflex Therapy*. New York: Creative Age.

SCHUTZ, W. C. (1967) *Joy*. New York: Grove Press.

SIDNEY, E. AND ARGYLE, M. (1969) *Training in Selection Interviewing*. London: Mantra.

SPIVACK, G. AND SHURE, M. B. (1974) *Social Adjustment of Young Children*. San Francisco, Cal.: Jossey Bass.

STAMPFL, T. G. AND LEVIS, D. J. (1967) Essentials of implosive therapy: a learning theory-based psychodynamic behavioral therapy. *Journal of Abnormal Psychology*, 72, 496–508.

TRUAX, C. B. AND CARKHUFF, R. R. (1967) *Toward Effective Counseling and Psychotherapy: Training and Practice*. Chicago, Ill.: Aldine.

VITALO, R. (1971) Teaching improved interpersonal functioning as a preferred mode of treatment. *Journal of Clinical Psychology*, 22, 166–71.

WELFORD, A. T. (1968) *Fundamentals of Skill*. London: Methuen.

WOLPE, J. (1958) *Psychotherapy by Reciprocal Inhibition*. Stanford, Cal.: Stanford University Press.

WOLPE, J. (1970) The instigation of assertive behavior: Transcripts from two cases. *Journal of Behavior Therapy and Experimental Psychiatry*. 1, 145–51.

WOLPE, J. (1973a) *The practice of behaviour therapy*. Oxford: Pergamon.

WOLPE, J. (1973b) Supervision Transcript V: Mainly about assertive training. *Journal of Behavior Therapy and Experimental Psychiatry*, 4, 141–8.

YATES, A. J. (1975) *Theory and Practice in Behavior Therapy*. New York: Wiley.

5 Outcome studies of skills training: a review

by John Marzillier

Does training in interpersonal skills work? If it does, what are the most efficient components of a skills training programme? In this chapter we shall look at the evidence. Before doing so, we will briefly consider the problems of experimental design in outcome research.

Experimental design

There are two basic ways in which the efficacy of a treatment can be systematically investigated. The first of these is to examine the effects on a single individual and this is often called a 'single case study'. This method has the advantages that treatment can be individually tailored to the patient's specific deficits and that clinical and research considerations can be combined without undue difficulty. It is, however, limited to conclusions which can be drawn from one patient, and it is rare in the literature to see unsuccessful single case studies described.

The second approach is to compare two or more groups of patients, one of which receives the experimental training and the others control treatments. This has the merit of seeing the effects on several patients, thereby allowing generalisations to be made with more confidence. In addition, various different sorts of comparisons can be made. Firstly, it is well known that patients can recover 'spontaneously' without any form of treatment, and the inclusion of a group who receives no treatment can take account of this. Secondly, it is also known that some patients respond to 'non-specific' aspects of treatment which are nothing to do with the particular treatment being given, such as receiving attention from a therapist or even taking a chalk pill, the so called 'placebo' effect. The inclusion of a control group of patients who receive an 'inactive' treatment can check on this, provided the inactive treatment constitutes a sensible alternative in which patients can believe; if it is too irrelevant it may simply be equivalent to no treatment. This may be very difficult to achieve, since almost any inactive treatment will provide opportunities for imitation and practice if it involves interaction with a skilled therapist or with other patients. Thirdly, patients may respond just as well to alternative, well-established treatments which may be cheaper, easier or quicker to administer, and one way of evaluating a new treatment is to show that it is as good as or superior to other treatments. Fourthly, different sorts of comparison can be made to evaluate the effects of different components of training itself, for example, whether modelling is better than practice or instruction.

The versatility of group designs has to be weighed against their disadvantages. The comparison of the *average* response to treatment of a group of patients can mask large individual variations within the group, concealing the fact that some patients may not have improved or may even have got worse. Moreover, standard training procedures and measures have to be used, and this leads to insensitivity to the needs of individual patients.

Social skills training is a complex treatment of complex problems, and because of this it does not lend itself easily to systematic experimental study of its effects. This is clear from the group studies to be reviewed in this chapter, many of which have design and measurement problems which indicate caution in accepting many reported results. In addition to the choice of sorts of groups, other problems arise mainly in the following areas:

1. *Length of treatment time.* All groups should have an equivalent amount of treatment time to ensure that differences between them cannot be attributed simply to the number of therapy hours. There are problems in this, in that some treatments,

such as insight therapy, inherently require more time than others, such as behavioural methods.

2. *Selection of subjects.* Groups should be similar or 'homogeneous' in the kinds of patients they contain, especially in terms of any factors likely to affect treatment, such as the level of their initial social defects. Homogeneity can theoretically be obtained by random allocation of patients to treatment groups, which has been done in most outcome studies, but this procedure is not always effective with small numbers, and many studies have, in fact, used small numbers of patients.

3. *Measures of change.* Because degrees of particular social qualities are not quantifiable in the way factors such as height, weight or temperature are, reliable and valid measurement of social behaviour is extremely difficult. Two main types of measurement have been used. (a) *Self-report measures*: these usually consist of questionnaires which invite the subject to say what he would feel or do in response to a hypothetical set of situations. Their main weakness is that it is not clear how reliable self-reported information is, nor how accurately it predicts behaviour. (b) *Ratings of observed behaviour*: many studies have incorporated standardised test situations in which the actual behaviour of the patient is observed and rated by a panel of judges. There is a danger of these tests becoming too artificial and one major, and by no means resolved, problem is ensuring that they are realistic and relevant to the individual's particular difficulties. Finally, as well as being reliable and valid, measures should be comprehensive. There has been a tendency in some studies to concentrate exclusively on social behaviour and ignore other important aspects of outcome such as clinical improvement.

4. *Generalisation and durability of change.* In addition to immediate improvements as a result of treatment, it has to be shown that changes generalise to life outside treatment, and that improvement is maintained over time. Some of the outcome measures should be designed to test social functioning in situations outside the clinic or laboratory, and follow-up assessments some months or even years after treatment should be included. This is probably the most difficult single problem in outcome studies.

5. *Therapist effects.* The success of a treatment may be influenced by the personal qualities (good or bad) of the therapist or

by his own beliefs in its efficacy. In comparing two treatments, therefore, bias may occur if the same therapist gives both treatments or if different therapists give different treatments. This can be partly avoided if at least two therapists are used, each of whom gives each treatment to a proportion of the patients. However, this can be costly, and it may be difficult for therapists of different persuasions to acquire each other's therapeutic skills in a short time.

6. *Additional therapies.* If patients taking part in a study are receiving other forms of therapy, such as drugs, in addition to the treatments being studied, this may affect the results, and ideally all other forms of treatment should be withheld for the duration of the experiment. This may not be possible for ethical reasons, particularly if a long follow-up period is incorporated, in which case these other therapies should be specified and controlled for. In only one of the studies to be reviewed was there any evidence that this had been done.

7. *'Contamination' of treatments.* The separate effects of two treatments can be obscured if patients discuss their respective treatments with each other or observe the other treatment in operation. This is most likely to occur with inpatients, and ideally the two treatments should be carried out on different wards or in different parts of the hospital.

8. *Independent assessment.* Outcome measures which involve ratings of behaviour should be made by independent judges who are ignorant of or 'blind' to the treatment received, so that their judgments are not influenced by their attitudes to either treatment. It is also preferable that they be ignorant of whether they are rating pre-treatment or post-treatment behaviour, but this is difficult to achieve unless different judges are used or unless all test behaviour can be filmed and randomly presented.

9. *Loss of subjects.* Even the most well-designed studies cannot protect themselves against subjects who do not stay the course. This may not be serious if losses occur for reasons unrelated to the treatment, such as death, physical illness or moving away. The effects are more serious if they occur as a result of aversive reactions to one or other treatment or, as may sometimes happen, due to the treatment being so successful that the patient no longer wishes to continue. In other words, if those who react worst (or best) to treatment drop out, the treatment may emerge

as more (or less) successful than it actually is. There is a temptation to keep the numbers in the study constant by replacing drop-outs with fresh patients, but this can introduce a similar bias.

Review of outcome research*

We have selected from a wide variety of studies those which are better designed and which meet the criteria of what constitutes skills training, namely to improve social behaviour by means of demonstration, practice, guidance and feedback.

For ease of presentation the studies on psychiatric patients have been divided into those done on inpatients and those done on outpatients, since the methods used and the results found in these two groups show important differences. With certain exceptions this division roughly corresponds to a division into studies of assertive training and studies of social skills training, or, again, into American studies and English studies. The inpatient studies have been further subdivided into those which attempt to evaluate the overall effects of skills training, and those which investigate the contribution of various components of a training programme. The outpatients studies were all of the former type.

A third section is concerned with studies done, not on patients, but on volunteer subjects. These studies have largely been concerned with the components of training, usually assertive training, and the majority of them were done in the U.S.A. They are included because of the contribution they may make to the development of skills training programmes for psychiatric patients.

STUDIES ON INPATIENTS

(a) *Effectiveness of skills training*
A number of well-designed studies on individual patients have demonstrated that skills training can improve social behaviour. Eisler, Hersen and Miller (1974) showed that assertive training consisting of instructions, role-playing and feedback improved the behaviour of two unassertive inpatients, in one case leading to substantial clinical improvement. Hersen *et al.* (1975) demonstrated that a social skills programme, in conjunction with

---

* Where improvements are reported, these are statistically significant unless otherwise stated.

pharmacological and industrial treatment, improved the conversation and assertive skills of a young male patient; this improvement was maintained at twenty-two weeks follow-up. Eisler (1976) assessed a similar social skills programme on the conversation skills of a middle-aged patient in his work environment. Training again led to specific improvements which were maintained three months later. Trower (1971) produced similar effects in a withdrawn male inpatient, but no follow-up was carried out. All these studies provide encouraging evidence for the efficacy of skills training on individual patients, but as single case studies they do not permit any general conclusions to be drawn.

More substantial conclusions can be drawn from control group studies. One of the best comparative studies on inpatients is that of Goldsmith and McFall (1975). This study compared the effects of a carefully compiled and realistic assertive training programme, an 'inactive' treatment, and no treatment. Ratings were made from patients' responses to two tests: a Behavioural Role-played Test consisting of twenty-five tape-recorded simulated interpersonal situations, and a conversation with a male confederate. Patients reported how comfortable and competent they felt themselves to be in these situations. This study also attempted to measure whether improvements generalised to situations outside treatment (by subdividing the interpersonal test situations into those used and not used in training), and also the long-term effects on re-admission rates eight months later.

The results showed that patients receiving training improved significantly on the two behavioural tests, as judged by independent raters and by themselves, while the patients in the two control groups did not. These improvements were also found in the situations not used in training, which indicates that some generalisation did occur. The long-term benefits of training could not be established as 28 per cent of the patients had been discharged or 'lost' at follow-up, but there was a trend towards a lower re-admission rate in the training group than the control group.

This study demonstrates that short-term improvements can be brought about by skills training. However, there were certain shortcomings in the design which should be mentioned. Perhaps the most important of these is the nature of the Behavioural Role-played Test. Since this particular test and versions of it have been used in many studies (see p. 120) it merits careful consideration. The presentation of a large number of tape-recorded situations has two advantages: (1) it can cover a wider range of situations than would be practical in 'live' presentations, and (2) it ensures that each subject undergoes an exactly comparable experience. Both of these are important factors in assessment, but their disadvantage is that they inevitably involve the sacrifice of any semblance of reality. It is very hard to imagine how responding to a tape-recorder can be considered 'interpersonal'. In Goldsmith and McFall's study the addition of the conversation test provided a useful check which has not always been used in other studies. Their test for generalisation effects, however, only included the simulated situations, and it is doubtful whether this can be said to be anything more than a 'technical' generalisation.

Another shortcoming of this study is that there was no attempt either to measure or to train non-verbal skills. There is evidence to suggest that non-verbal signals which convey warmth and rewardingness are of great importance in 'toning down' the aggressive component of assertion (see chapter 3).

Gutride, Goldstein and Hunter (1973, 1974) carried out two studies on acute and chronic inpatients to assess a form of social skills training which they called Structured Learning Therapy. This comprised videotaped demonstrations of ways of initiating and responding to conversation, coaching in important aspects which related to individual difficulties, practice and videotaped feedback, and social reinforcement. The therapy was given in group form and the group met three times a week for four weeks. Ratings of behaviour were made from a structured test situation and from observations at mealtimes in the hospital.

The first study showed structured learning therapy to produce a significant improvement in both acute and chronic patients compared with a no-treatment control group. However there was a substantial loss of patients, and some design faults – for instance, the behavioural assessment was made only after treatment and no follow up of long-term effects was included.

The second study added an inactive treatment control group, and also included a transfer training programme, in which patients were given an extra two weeks' treatment in the hospital dining room. The results showed structured learning therapy to be superior to both the inactive treatment and the no-treatment control groups in improving behaviour in the structured test situation but not in the dining room. The addition of transfer training failed to show any greater effect than training on its own, a disappointing result since this is one of very few studies which has attempted to provide training in a 'natural' setting. Clinical and follow-up assessments were not included.

These studies by Goldsmith and McFall and Gutride *et al.* are probably the best-designed studies on inpatients which attempt to evaluate the overall effectiveness of skills training. They do show that training can produce improvements in behaviour in a hospital setting, even with chronic patients, but they have not successfully demonstrated that these effects last, nor that they generalise to real-life situations. Furthermore, it is not clear that they were of clinical benefit to the patients.

It is not possible to review all the studies which have been done on inpatients, but many of them have produced more equivocal results or have contained design faults which make their interpretation difficult (Lomont, Gilner, Spector and Skinner 1969; Ullrich de Muynck and Ullrich 1972; Serber and Nelson 1971; Rivlin 1974; Vitalo 1971).

(b) *Evaluation of components of skills training*

A number of studies have been concerned with the relative contribution of various components of skills training, such as demonstration, guidance and practice, to changing the behaviour of inpatients.

Goldstein *et al.* (1973) investigated the effects of different types of models on assertive behaviour. They found that patients who listened to tape-recordings of an 'independent' (assertive) model responding to a number of frustrating or threatening social situations subsequently gave more assertive responses themselves than patients who listened to an unassertive model or who had no model presented. However, no assessment was made of transfer to real-life situations, no follow-up was made and non-verbal behaviour was not included.

Hersen, Eisler and Miller conducted a series of experiments comparing the effects of modelling and other components of training on increasing assertive behaviour. The main measure of change in all these experiments consisted of asking the patient to respond to five simulated interpersonal situations requiring assertive responses. It was thus similar to the test used by Goldsmith and McFall, although it contained fewer situations. On the other hand, it broadened the scope of assessment and training to include non-verbal as well as verbal behaviour, by using videotapes rather than audiotapes both to present the situations and to record the patient's responses. Patients receiving treatment were given four treatment sessions and then reassessed, while a control group simply carried out both assessments without intervening treatment. The whole process of assessment and treatment took only three days.

In the first study (Eisler, Hersen and Miller 1973), modelling was shown to be superior to practice in increasing assertive behaviour. Patients in the practice group did not do any better than the no-treatment control groups. In a subsequent study, Hersen, Eisler, Miller, Johnson and Pinkston (1973) assessed the contribution of a further component, 'instructions', which consisted of asking patients to concentrate on certain aspects of the interaction – for example, talking, or looking at the other person, for a longer time. The results again showed modelling to be superior, either alone, or in conjunction with instructions. Instructions alone, however, were more effective in increasing loudness of speech, whereas in the previous study modelling had had most effect.

In a third study by Hersen, Eisler and Miller (1974), two further dimensions were added to assess generalisation effects. Some patients received the additional instruction to apply what they had learned to new situations, and all patients were given a generalisation task which consisted of the experimenter failing to give a promised monetary reward for participation in the study. The results again confirmed the superiority of modelling and instruction, but the group receiving 'instructions to generalise' fared no better than other training groups. Indeed the experiment failed to show any generalisation effects, since *none* of the treatments produced a significant improvement on the generalisation task.

Hersen and his colleagues claim that their studies provide some information about the effective components of training programmes. In particular, modelling, either alone or in combination with instructions, consistently emerged as superior, while practice repeatedly failed to effect change. However, the modelling effect was limited to the five simulated situations and did not generalise to the real-life test. On reflection this is not, perhaps, surprising, given the brevity of the treatment and the fact that assessment and training were concentrated on the same situations, since the process of imitation involves not just straightforward copying or rote learning of responses, but also the induction of of rules which can be applied to a range of similar situations. By the same token, 'instructions to generalise' – i.e. the mere telling of someone to apply what they had learned – would be unlikely to succeed if the underlying rules had not, in fact, been acquired.

It would also be unfortunate to assume from these results that practice is irrelevant. No feedback was given to patients, and we have seen in the previous chapter that practice is most likely to be effective with knowledge of results. Furthermore, the training was extremely brief and may not have allowed enough time for practice to take effect.

Finally, because of the lack of follow-up assessment and the uncertain clinical relevance of responses to pre-selected, simulated interpersonal situations, we should be cautious about drawing any definite conclusions from these studies.

(c) *Summary of inpatient studies*

These studies provide encouraging evidence that, at least in the short term, skills training can produce improvements in behaviour and subjective feelings of comfort in social situations, sometimes within a very short period of time, and on patients with widely differing diagnoses including acute and chronic schizophrenia, neuroses and personality disorders.

Against this it must be said that some of the changes reported have been very limited, and that there is no evidence that these changes either lasted or helped patients to cope with real-life situations. Nor have they been shown to be of benefit to patients in alleviating distressing clinical symptoms. Furthermore, there is little information on the differential effects of training on different kinds of patients and problems. Only chronic versus acute patients were compared, and no research has yet looked systematically at such major variables as diagnosis, social class, age, sex and I.Q.

As far as components of training are concerned, there is evidence that modelling and instruction are useful techniques for inpatients. There was no evidence on the effectiveness of giving feedback, and video feedback was not commonly used, although this has been found useful in other areas.

STUDIES ON OUTPATIENTS

One advantage of skills training for outpatients is that social life has not been disrupted by admission to hospital, and patients can therefore practise new skills as they are learned in a wide range of normal social encounters. However, this can also be a disadvantage, since the experimenter has no control over events outside treatment, cannot easily observe what goes on and must rely on patients' own accounts of their experiences.

Relatively few investigations of skills training have been carried out on outpatients; these have largely been concerned with the overall effects of training rather than with the evaluation of its components.

Wolpe (1958, 1973), reported a substantial degree of success using assertive training on neurotic outpatients. Similarly, a number of case studies have been reported in which assertive training, either alone or in conjunction with other therapies, proved beneficial on a variety of outpatient problems (Bloomfield 1973; Goldstein, Serber and Piaget 1970; Newman 1969). Lazarus (1966) reported a favourable outcome for behaviour rehearsal in comparison with a non-directive therapy, but since he carried out all the treatment and assessment himself, the results are rather suspect.

A few single case studies have looked at the effects of training on more specific clinical problems. Eisler and his colleagues produced beneficial effects in marital interaction (Eisler, Miller, Hersen and Jackson 1974) and family interaction (Eisler and Hersen 1973), and in a case of 'explosive rages' (Foy and Eisler, in press). Hallam (1974) used skills training with an extinction schedule to eliminate rituals in an obsessional patient. Barlow, Agras and Reynolds (1972) and Yardley (in press) used skills training to increase gender-appropriate behaviour in transsexuals. Qualified transfer of training was reported in all these cases, but they were not all properly controlled single case studies.

Two control group studies on the effect of social skills training on outpatients were carried out by the authors. In our first study (Argyle, Bryant and Trower 1974) we compared social skills training in individual form with psychotherapy. Sixteen patients were assessed after a three-week period of no treatment to allow for stabilisation of medication, and then randomly assigned to one treatment. The two treatment groups were also subdivided into those who received treatment immediately and those who were on a six-week waiting list and thus acted as a no-treatment control. Patients were in treatment for an equal period of time, six weeks, but the psychotherapy patients received three sessions a week while the training patients received only one. This was done on the grounds that these were appropriate lengths of time, given the nature and purpose of each treatment, and any bias operating would be in favour of the control treatment.

The social skills training comprised modelling, instruction, practice and videotape feedback, with homework assignments carried out between sessions. The main dependent measures were a behavioural test involving a ten-minute interaction with a stranger, from which elements of social performance (e.g. volume of speech, facial expression, gaze, speech content) were rated by independent judges, and a self-report questionnaire of the amount of difficulty experienced in thirty everyday situations.

The results showed that both treatments tended to be effective in improving behavioural skills compared with no treatment, and both groups reported less difficulty and fewer feelings of in-competence. However, at six-week follow-up the gains on the self-report measures made by the patients receiving social skills training persisted more strongly than for the patients receiving psychotherapy. This was only a trend to statistical significance, although at six month follow-up this trend was supported by lower re-referral rates in the training group.

Better results for social skills training might have been achieved if patients had received more training; six one-hour sessions do not allow a great deal of time. Also, the fact that the psychotherapy patients received three times as much treatment may have biased the results against the experimental treatment, and a fairer com-parison may have been to have equated the amount of time spent in treatment.

In our second study (Trower et al., in press) we compared social skills training with modified systematic desensitisation for twenty socially inadequate outpatients. Patients were selected on the basis of standard criteria of social inadequacy (see chapter 3), were randomly allocated to treatment and to one of two therapists, and were each given ten individual sessions. The assessments were similar to those used in the previous study, except that the behavioural test was refined to tap a range of skills, such as listening, speaking and assertive skills and conversation management. All assessments, including the behavioural test, were repeated six months after treatment. Follow-up assessments were made at one, three and six months after treatment.

On the clinical measures, both treatments led to a reduction in symptoms of anxiety, depression and social phobia. On the behavioural measures the results were mixed. Total scores on a rating scale and on quantitative measures showed no significant change in either treatment group. However, quantitative measures of patients' worst individual deficits showed both treatments to be effective on general items and social skills training to be superior to desensitisation on more specific ones. On the self-report measures social skills training reduced the amount of difficulty reported and increased the amount of social activities entered into, while desensitisation did not. These improvements were maintained, and indeed increased during the follow-up period. The training group also had less non-experimental treatment during this period.*

Marzillier, Lambert and Kellett (1976) carried out a similar study comparing social skills training with systematic desensitisation and with a no-treatment control on twenty-one psychiatric outpatients who complained of major social difficulties. Social skills training consisted of modelling, role-playing and audio-taped feedback, with homework assignments between sessions. Desensitisation was carried out in the traditional manner supplemented by 'in vivo' practice where necessary. Patients in both treatment groups were seen individually by one therapist who carried out all the treatment. Treatment was over an average of $3\frac{1}{2}$ months for a maximum of fifteen once weekly sessions. Patients in the control group were told they were on a waiting list and were reassessed after $3\frac{1}{2}$ months before going on to receive treatment.

The outcome measures included a behavioural test consisting of a videotaped brief conversation with a female stranger, from which independent ratings of conversational skills, social anxiety and 'general ability to cope' were made. Other measures were

* But this finding was not significant.

target rating scales, social anxiety questionnaires and a diary of social activities and contacts. The latter were also used to assess patients six months later.

The major finding was that patients in all groups, including the no-treatment group, improved on most measures. The two treatment groups showed greater improvement on the social diary measure than the no-treatment group. At six-months follow-up only patients in the social skills training group provided a sufficient number of returns for statistical analysis; the gains made by these patients was maintained.

The authors report some problems in this study which make interpretation of the results difficult. Therapist and treatment effects were confounded by the use of only one therapist. There were practical difficulties in implementing both treatments. Some patients in the social skills training group had difficulty in transferring skills learned in treatment to real-life situations. Some patients in the desensitisation group had difficulty in imagining scenes realistically, while others found it impossible to achieve a reasonable state of relaxation, and this group was badly depleted by drop-outs, suggesting possible adverse responses to this form of treatment.

A further problem in this study and the present authors' second study was the absence of an inactive therapy control group. Without this it is not possible definitely to attribute improvements found equally in both treatments to the specific effects of either treatment, since they might be the result of the non-specific effect of being in treatment.

Summary of outpatient studies

The three main control group studies on outpatients show that social skills training can produce improvements in general social functioning. These improvements seemed to be lasting ones, at least over the follow-up period. The training also appeared to be of clinical benefit, and to make a real contribution towards expanding the social life of the patients and reducing their need for further treatment.

Against this, the three studies were unable to establish any very clearcut behavioural changes in favour of social skills training, and patients appeared to benefit clinically as much from desensitisation as from social skills training.

CONCLUSIONS FOR PSYCHIATRIC PATIENTS

Taking the inpatient and outpatient studies together, what can we conclude about the effectiveness of skills training for psychiatric patients?

First, there is evidence that skills training can improve *behavioural skills*. The clearest support for this comes from the inpatient studies which were, with the exception of Gutride's, largely concerned with assertive training rather than social skills training. It is possible that the more limited nature and aims of assertive training make it easier to devise specific training and outcome measures, and therefore to show changes.

Furthermore, inpatients are likely to be more disturbed than outpatients, which would imply that their behavioural deficits would be more extreme. It is always easier to measure gross deficits and changes from extreme to less extreme than from fairly bad to better. This may explain why Gutride, whose structured learning therapy was very similar in many ways to our social skills training, was able to show clear behavioural improvements on acute and chronic patients, including schizophrenics, while the outpatient studies only found limited behavioural changes. On the other hand inpatients, especially chronic ones, are generally thought to be less responsive to treatment.

Another reason why the inpatient studies may have been more successful in demonstrating the superiority of skills training is that control treatments used were all 'inactive' therapies which, by definition, were not expected to change behaviour. In the outpatient studies, on the other hand, the control treatments were not only 'active' but were chosen because of their relevance to the problem. They may thus have been indirectly improving social skills – desensitisation through reducing anxiety in social situations and encouraging covert rehearsal, and psychotherapy through the exploration of motives and social relationships. This might explain why social skills did not emerge as definitely superior to the control treatment, but does not account for the fact that none of the treatments in the outpatient studies appeared to produce very obvious changes in behaviour.

Second, there is evidence that the effects of training *generalise* to real life and are of *lasting* benefit. This evidence comes from the studies of social skills training on outpatients, and was not found in the inpatient studies.

We suggest that there may be several reasons why generalisation effects were not found in the inpatient studies: (1) the extreme brevity of the assertive training given to inpatients; (2) the artificial nature of the assertive training which comprised responses to recorded conversations and not to 'live' interactions; (3) the opportunities which outpatients have throughout treatment to practise their skills in real life; (4) the broader nature of social skills training (given to the outpatients) which encourages patients to conceptualise social rules which can be applied to a range of situations. If this is so, it is not clear why Gutride's structured learning therapy failed to show any generalisation effects, since the treatment was of a reasonable length and involved 'live' interactions. One possible explanation is that the 'real life' of these patients in hospital would largely involve interaction with other patients who might themselves be socially inadequate. It is possible, therefore, that the improved social skills of the training patients would fail to evoke the rewarding responses from fellow patients which they might have got from 'normal' people, thereby not reinforcing the patients' attempts.

Evidence for generalisation effects in the outpatient studies came mainly from the patients' own reports of their activities and difficulty (though this does not apply to re-referral rates), and it is a problem to know how accurate they were. It is possible that they were exaggerated after treatment, perhaps out of a desire to please the therapists. However, if this were so it should apply equally to both treatments, and our second study clearly showed these improvements to be only for the social skills training patients.

Third, there is evidence that skills training is of *clinical* benefit to patients; this again comes from the outpatient studies of social skills training. One reason why the inpatient studies did not show clinical improvement is that most of them did not look for it. Goldsmith and McFall did include re-admission rates at follow-up but this is a rather crude clinical measure. In fact, the extreme brevity of the assertive training would suggest that substantial clinical improvement would have been rather unlikely. It is a pity that Gutride's more lengthy training was not assessed for clinical outcome.

The importance of including clinical measure was demonstrated in a study by Vitalo (1971) which compared training in qualities of warmth, genuineness and empathy with traditional group therapy. The results showed the training to be superior to group therapy on measures of social behaviour. On clinical measures, however, it did not fare so well. Only the group therapy patients showed significant reductions in clinical disturbance, and, moreover, the training produced a significant *increase* in anxiety. Thus, although the training programme produced predicted improvement in interpersonal skills, the patients receiving training appeared to be clinically worse off than those who received traditional group therapy.

It should be noted that the clinical improvements found in the outpatient studies were not confined to social skills training, but were also found in the control treatments, and in Marzillier's study the no-treatment group also improved. We cannot, therefore, definitely attribute the clinical improvement to the treatments.

Finally, while we believe these studies on psychiatric patients are encouraging, there have been too few of them, and probably as many questions have been raised as answered. Further studies are needed before any firm claims can be made about the efficiency of skills training.

STUDIES ON VOLUNTEER SUBJECTS

More studies have been conducted on volunteer subjects than on inpatients and outpatients combined. Most of them have been concerned with evaluating the contribution of various components of training, and in this sense they may be useful in developing treatment for psychiatric patients. However, it should not necessarily be assumed that the results found in volunteer studies can be uncritically applied to patients. In the first place, the volunteer subjects used in these studies are almost invariably college students whose degree of deficit is likely to be less than that of patients. Secondly, the students often received credits towards their study courses as a reward for participation which suggests that they were highly motivated towards treatment. This may increase the chances of obtaining successful results compared with less motivated patients. With this caution in mind we will briefly review the main volunteer studies.

McFall and his colleagues carried out several studies evaluating the effectiveness of components of assertive training. The format of all these studies was basically the same. Their chief outcome measure was the Behavioural Role-played Test of assertiveness described earlier (p. 109). Other measures included a Conflict Resolution Inventory which comprised responses to a list of 35 situations requiring refusal to unreasonable requests and 8 items of a more general nature. They also included a follow-up assessment in the form of a telephone call by a confederate of the experimenter who made an 'unreasonable' request.

In the first study (McFall and Marston 1970), practice with and without tape-recorded feedback was compared with an inactive treatment and with no treatment in an automated four-session programme. The subjects were forty-two unassertive college students. The results showed that the two practice treatments combined were superior to the control groups in increasing assertive behaviour, in contrast to the findings of Eisler and his colleagues with psychiatric patients (reviewed above). Partial support for this result was also reported on the telephone follow-up test.

The second study (McFall and Lillesand 1971) evaluated the effects of two additional components, modelling and coaching, combined with either 'overt' rehearsal (a verbal response which was played back to the subject) or 'covert' (silent) rehearsal. The results showed that after only two training sessions both treatments were superior to a no-treatment control group, but these results were not found in the telephone follow-up test. There were no significant differences between the treatments, but a tendency for covert rehearsal to show the greater change. The separate contribution of modelling and coaching was not assessed.

In an attempt to resolve some of the ambiguities, McFall and Twentyman (1973) studied the contribution of modelling, coaching and covert rehearsal in two separate studies. The first study showed all combinations of training components to be effective compared with a no-treatment control. Covert rehearsal alone was less effective than rehearsal with coaching, but the addition of modelling did not appear to make any difference. The telephone follow-up test showed no treatment effects, which the authors attributed to a poor choice of request which may not have been sufficiently unreasonable. The second study, which was very similar to the first, replicated these results.

In a third experiment, McFall and Twentyman found that

neither a more tactful model nor the presentation of the model on videotape rather than audiotape enhanced the modelling effect. In addition, a comparison of covert and overt rehearsal showed no significant differences.

These experiments demonstrate that a brief, standardised training programme can increase assertive behaviour in the short term. The best combination of techniques appeared to be rehearsal and coaching, and modelling did not appear to contribute anything further. However, as McFall and Twentyman point out, the student subjects in these experiments were probably not completely lacking in assertive skills to start with, and modelling may be more influential with individuals who are deficient in basic assertive skills. The studies of Eisler, Hersen and Miller suggest that some form of modelling may be essential for psychiatric patients.

In contrast to McFall and Twentyman's results, Friedman (1971) did find an incremental effect for modelling, in that combined modelling and role-playing was superior to role-playing alone. However, there were some problems with this study. Friedman's main outcome measure was a behavioural test which comprised only one situation, and ratings made from this test were not very reliable.

In the McFall and Friedman studies a very limited amount of training was carried out over a very short time. Rathus (1972, 1973) evaluated the effects of a programme spanning several weeks, which is closer to the studies of social skills training on psychiatric patients. The two main outcome measures were a standardised assertiveness questionnaire and a structured interview in which subjects were asked to say what they would do in various situations requiring assertiveness. The first study compared assertive training in group form to group discussion of fear. On the assertiveness questionnaire both treatments were found to be effective; in the structured interview, greater improvement was found for the training group, but this was not maintained. The second study added videotaped examples of assertive behaviour to the training, and the control treatment consisted of observation of a film showing a girl receiving systematic desensitisation for social fears. Assertive training was found to be superior to the control treatment on both outcome measures.

A major weakness of these two studies was that the actual

behaviour of the subjects was not assessed. Also the control treatments were not very appropriate. In the first study the control group discussed fear and not assertiveness, so a direct comparison of training versus discussion was not possible. The observation of filmed desensitisation used in the second study would appear to be somewhat irrelevant to the acquisition of assertive skills, and it is hardly surprising that it failed to show any effect. A further limitation was the lack of data on the subjects' initial inadequacy.

The contribution of positive social reinforcement (i.e. praising appropriate responses) was examined in a study by Young, Rimm and Kennedy (1973). The results showed that social reinforcement did not result in more assertive behaviour than modelling without reinforcement. However, this may have been due to the population studied with comprised students whose degree of unassertiveness was not clearly established. Clinical applications of assertive training incorporate a substantial element of social reinforcement, as a study of Wolpe's indicates (Wolpe 1970). Where assertive responses are markedly deficient, social or other reinforcement procedures may well be important.

In an interesting study by Thorpe (1975), self-instructional training, in which subjects were required to rehearse more productive cognitions first out loud and then silently, was found to be equal to or better than assertive training. No significant differences were found on measures of generalisation or a telephone follow-up assessment.

The importance of cognitive processes was also highlighted by Kazdin (1974), who showed that an entirely 'imagined' treatment could produce changes in behaviour. In this study, which used the behavioural role-played test devised by McFall and Lillesand, one group of subjects imagined an assertive model, while another group in addition imagined favourable consequences arising out of the model's behaviour. The results showed both methods to be effective, including self-reported improvement at three-months follow-up, but the group which imagined favourable consequences did even better. Both groups were equally effective on the generalisation items of the test. The telephone follow-up failed to show any differences between treatments, but this result was complicated by the fact that the treatment groups also did not differ from a group of people randomly selected from the telephone directory.

Summary of volunteer studies

These studies on volunteer students provide evidence that assertive training can increase assertiveness in the short term, often in a very short period of time. In this they are similar to the studies on inpatients.

They differ from the inpatient studies in that practice was found to be effective, even if it was silent rather than acted out, and modelling was not found, in some studies, to be useful.

Some volunteer studies suggest that cognitive processes are important, in that changing the subject's cognition by getting him simply to imagine an assertive model can increase assertiveness. The processes involved are not clear, but it is possible that in order to imagine a successful model, as opposed to having it provided, the subject has first to work out some of the rules underlying successful behaviour.

On the debit side, a weakness of the volunteer studies, as with the inpatient studies, was their failure to show that changes either endure or generalise beyond treatment. In fact most of the studies appeared to confuse these two aspects. Follow-up assessments consisted almost entirely of contrived telephone calls which were often made after only a short period and sometimes after only a few days. They cannot therefore be said to measure long-term effects.

Furthermore, the telephone calls introduced a new situation quite different from those used in assessment or training, and in this sense they would appear to test for generalisation rather than follow-up effects. In fact the calls were the only tests of generalisation which attempted to measure a real-life situation, since most other tests were simulated situations like those used in treatment. In this sense the telephone calls failed to demonstrate convincingly that the effects of training generalised as they were usually unsuccessful. In one study it was felt that the test had failed because the particular request may have seemed reasonable and would not, therefore, have been refused. While this may be so, the persistent failure of these tests in most studies may well indicate that generalisation was not occurring. We have already discussed some possible reasons for this (see p. 118).

The failure to incorporate proper follow-up assessments is a serious one, as was illustrated in a study by Hedquist and Weinhold (1970). Treatment effects were noted to decline towards the end of treatment, and at two-weeks follow-up the treatment groups were not significantly different from a control group.

A further weakness in many of the volunteer studies is the failure to establish any specific criteria of unassertiveness. Some studies suggest that subjects already possessed some basic assertive skills, which would seem likely among normal college students, and were being instigated to greater assertiveness rather than being taught the rudiments. It is not entirely clear, therefore, how far some of the results are appropriate to psychiatric patients, especially inpatients, whose deficits are more serious. It should not be assumed too readily that methods seen to be promising with students will necessarily be successful on patients until replicated on patients.

Discussion

It is only in the last few years that training methods for treating social problems have developed to any degree. As in any new development, it is difficult to discriminate clear evidence for the effectiveness of skills training until a substantial body of research has been carried out. It is also difficult to sift the available evidence to discern which components of a complex treatment may be the most important ones in producing beneficial changes. These problems are very much in evidence in this review of training methods. Nevertheless, some general conclusions can be drawn from the studies and suggestions made for future developments in this field.

1. Experimental evidence from studies on both psychiatric patients and volunteer subjects indicates that skills training can produce positive changes in social behaviour in the short term. In the better designed studies it has been shown that this is not due to chance factors, nor to the non-specific effects of treatment.

2. Most of this evidence for behavioural change comes from studies of assertive training. These studies have failed to show that improvements are maintained over time, or that they help individuals to cope with real-life situations. Assertive training with psychiatric patients has not been shown to be of clinical benefit to patients in other respects. One explanation of these failures is that measures used to assess long-term, generalisation and clinical

effects were inadequate, or omitted altogether. On the other hand, these failures may reflect limitation of training programmes which are extremely brief, highly specific and somewhat artificial. Only further research can establish which explanation is correct.

3. Studies of social skills training on outpatients showed only limited effects on changing behaviour. This may have been due to inadequacies in the training which is more broadly based and less specific. On the other hand, two studies did show some behaviour changes in favour of training, and it may be that the effects of a more generalised training are more difficult to measure. In contrast to the assertive training studies, the outpatient studies provided some evidence that the improvements appeared to be of lasting benefit, and that they helped patients to enjoy a more extensive and satisfying social life. Social skills training was also found to improve clinical state at least as much as established control treatments.

4. Since the outpatient studies all involved social skills training, and the inpatient studies largely involved assertive training, it is not possible to disentangle the effects of the type of training and the type of patient. Further research is needed in this respect.

5. The different training and measurement techniques of the assertive training and social skills training studies may reflect a different choice of priorities in the English and American approaches. Both approaches are firmly committed to scientific evaluation and to meeting the requirements of experimental design, but the American studies have, we believe, generally ended up being too rigid in their methods, with a subsequent loss in appropriateness and relevance to daily life. The English studies have been more flexible in tempering experimental with real-life considerations, resulting in some loss of rigour but more meaning-fulness in both the content of training and measurements of outcome.

6. The components of a successful training programme have not been clearly established, as there has been too little evidence bearing on this question. Modelling and practice have been the subject of most experimental investigation. There is some sugges-tion that for subjects who already have a basic repertoire of assertive skills, modelling may not be necessary and practice is more relevant. However, for those who are severely deficient in such skills, modelling may well be essential. For psychiatric

patients the balance of evidence is in favour of incorporating some form of modelling into the treatment programme.

7. Finally, in reviewing these outcome studies we have drawn attention to a number of design problems and to the fact that some results have been rather inconclusive. While we believe that a critical approach is healthy, it should be remembered that from a statistical point of view the risks of accepting a false difference have to be balanced against the risks of rejecting a true difference. Thus, although flaws in experimental design suggest the need for caution in accepting too readily any results which demonstrate the efficacy of skills training, the same design faults can also conceal true differences in its favour. The studies done so far, taken together, are encouraging, but point to the need for better designs and measures in a field which is proving to be very difficult and yet extremely promising.

FUTURE RESEARCH NEEDS

A priority in future research is to establish methods of maintaining new behaviour and generalising it to real life. Kazdin (1975) has suggested seven ways that these might be achieved. (1) Rewards which normally occur in the environment should be used in training, so that new behaviour will have the same reinforcing consequences outside the training situation. (2) Individuals in the patient's environment can be trained to reward him in appropriate ways. (3) When new skills are well established, training sessions and the attendant support can be lessened gradually rather than abruptly, and (4) rewards can be 'thinned' or 'intermittent', a technique well-established in operant research. (5) New behaviour can be developed in a variety of situations and in the presence of several individuals. (6) New behaviour may be maintained by gradually increasing the delay between an appropriate response and its reward, for instance by increasing praise at the end of a sequence or session and decreasing it after each response. (7) Patients can be taught to evaluate their own behaviour and set their own criteria for rewarding themselves. The patient then becomes in control of events rather than being controlled by others. Some of these techniques already form part of our social skills training described in the second part of the book.

A second important area for future research is further investigation into the various components of training. This should be done on subjects who are representative of those for whom the training is intended, either patients themselves or volunteers whose social difficulties are very similar to those of patients. The focus of such investigations should be on the importance of different types of modelling, role-playing and feedback. It would be particularly useful to establish the importance of videotapes for modelling and feedback in comparison with audiotapes or other methods (Griffiths 1974), since this specialised equipment is very costly. More attention should also be paid to cognitive processes, and the extent to which training can improve the individual's ability to induce rules of social behaviour.

Finally, more research is needed on the characteristics of patients who would be suitable for various training approaches. So far, few outcome studies have attempted to compare the response to training of groups distinguished on such characteristics as the type of behavioural deficit, personality, diagnosis, social class, age, sex, and I.Q.

References

ARGYLE, M., BRYANT, B. M. AND TROWER, P. E. (1974) Social skills training and psychotherapy: a comparative study. *Psychological Medicine*, 4, 435–43.

BARLOW, D. H., AGRAS, W. AND REYNOLDS, J. (1972) Direct and indirect modification of specific motor behavior in a transsexual. 80th Annual Meeting, American Psychological Association, September, Honolulu, Hawaii.

BLOOMFIELD, H. H. (1973) Assertive training in an outpatient group of chronic schizophrenics: a preliminary report. *Behavior Therapy*, 4, 277–81.

EISLER, R. M. (1976) Assertive training in the work situation. In Krumboltz, J. and Thoresen, E. E. (eds) *Behavioral Counseling Methods*. New York: Holt, Rinehart & Winston.

EISLER, R. M. AND HERSEN, M. (1973) Behavioral techniques in family-oriented crisis intervention. *Archives General Psychiatry*, 28, 111–16.

EISLER, R. M., HERSEN, M. AND MILLER, P. M. (1973) Effects of modeling on components of assertive behavior. *Journal of Behavioral Therapy and Experimental Psychiatry*, 4, 1–6.

EISLER, R. M., HERSEN, M. AND MILLER, P. M. (1974) Shaping components of assertive behavior with instructions and feedback. *American Journal of Psychiatry*, 131, 1344–7.

EISLER, R. M., MILLER, P. M. AND HERSEN, M. (1973) Components of assertive behavior. *Journal of Clinical Psychology*, 29, 295–9.

EISLER, R. M., MILLER, P. M., HERSEN, M. AND JACKSON, H. A. (1974) Effects of assertive training on marital interaction. *Archives of General Psychiatry*, 30, 643–9.

FITTS, P. M. AND POSNER, M. I. (1967) *Human Performance*. Monterey, S. Calif.: Brooks/Cole.

FOY, D. W. AND EISLER, R. M. (in press) Modeled assertion in a case of explosive rages. *Journal of Behavior Therapy and Experimental Psychiatry*.

FRIEDMAN, P. H. (1971) The effects of modeling and role-playing in assertive behavior. In Rubin *et al.* (eds) *Advances in Behavior Therapy*. New York: Academic Press.

GOLDSMITH, JEAN, B. AND MCFALL, R. M. (1975) Development and evaluation of an interpersonal skill-training program for psychiatric in-patients. *Journal of Abnormal Psychology*, 84, 57–8.

GOLDSTEIN, A. P., MARTENS, J., HUBBEN, J., VAN BELLE, H. A., SCHAAF, W., WIERSMA, H. AND GOEDHART, A. (1973) The use of modeling to increase independent behavior. *Behaviour Research and Therapy*, 11, 31–42.

GOLDSTEIN, A. J., SERBER, M. AND PIAGET, G. (1970) Induced anger as a reciprocal inhibitor of fear. *Journal of Behavior Therapy and Experimental Psychiatry*, 1, 67–70.

GRIFFITHS, R. D. P. (1974) Videotape feedback as a therapeutic technique: Retrospect and prospect. *Behaviour Research and Therapy*, 12, 1–8.

GUTRIDE, M. E., GOLDSTEIN, A. P. AND HUNTER, G. F. (1973) The use of modeling and role-playing to increase social interaction among asocial psychiatric patients. *Journal of Consulting and Clinical Psychology*, 400, 408–15.

GUTRIDE, M. E., GOLDSTEIN, A. P. AND HUNTER, G. R. (1974) The use of structured learning therapy and transfer training in the treatment of chronic psychiatric patients. *Journal of Clinical Psychology*, 30, 277–80.

HALLAM, R. S. (1974) Extinction of ruminations: A case study. *Behavior Therapy*, 5, 565–8.

HEDQUIST, F. J. AND WEINHOLD, B. K. (1970) Behavioral group counseling with socially anxious and unassertive college students. *Journal of Counseling Psychology*, 17, 237–42.

HERSEN, M., EISLER, R. M. AND MILLER, P. (1974) An experimental analysis of generalisation in assertive training. *Behaviour Research and Therapy*, 12, 295–310.

HERSEN, M., EISLER, R. M., MILLER, P. M., JOHNSON, M. B. AND PINKSTON, S. G. (1973) Effects of practice, instructions and modeling on components of assertive behavior. *Behaviour Research and Therapy*, 11, 443–5.

HERSEN, M., TURNER, S. M., EDELSTEIN, B. A. AND PINKSTON, S. G. (1975) Effects of phenothiazines and social skills training in a withdrawn schizophrenic. *Journal of Clinical Psychology*, 31, 588–94.

KAZDIN, A. E. (1974) Effects of covert modeling and model reinforcement on assertive behavior. *Journal of Abnormal Psychology*, 83, 240–52.

Outcome studies of skills training: a review 129

KAZDIN, A. E. (1975) *Behavior Modification in Applied Settings.* Homewood, Ill.: The Dorsey Press.

LAZARUS, A. A. (1966) Behavior rehearsal versus non-directive therapy versus advice in effecting behavioral change. *Behaviour Research and Therapy* 4, 209–12.

LOMONT, J. F., GILNER, F. H., SPECTOR, N. J. AND SKINNER, K. K. (1969) Group assertion training and group insight therapies. *Psychonomic Science,* 25, 463–70.

MCFALL, R. M. AND LILLESAND, D. (1971) Behavior rehearsal with modeling and coaching in assertive training. *Journal of Abnormal Psychology,* 77, 313–23.

MCFALL, R. M. AND MARSTON, A. R. (1970) An experimental investigation of behavior rehearsal in assertive training. *Journal of Abnormal Psychology,* 76, 295–303.

MCFALL, R. M. AND TWENTYMAN, C. T. (1973) Four experiments on the relative contribution of rehearsal, modeling and coaching to assertion training. *Journal of Abnormal Psychology,* 81, 199–218.

MARZILLIER, J. S., LAMBERT, C. AND KELLETT, J. (1976) A controlled evaluation of systematic desensitization and social skills training for socially inadequate psychiatric patients. *Behaviour Research and Therapy,* 14, 225–38.

NEWMAN, D. (1969) Using assertive training. In Krumboltz, J. D. and Thorensen, C. E. (eds) *Behavioral Counseling: Cases and Techniques.* New York: Holt, Rinehart & Winston.

RATHUS, S. A. (1972) An experimental investigation of assertive training in a group setting. *Journal of Behavior Therapy and Experimental Psychiatry,* 3, 81–6.

RATHUS, S. A. (1973) Instigation of assertive behavior through videotape-mediated assertive models and directed practice. *Behaviour Research and Therapy,* 11, 57–65.

RIVLIN, E. (1974) A social skills approach to the treatment of clinical depression. Unpublished M. Phil. dissertation, University of London.

SERBER, M. AND NELSON, P. (1971) The ineffectiveness of systematic desensitization and assertive training in hospitalized schizophrenics. *Journal of Behavior Therapy and Experimental Psychiatry,* 2, 107–9.

THORPE, G. L. (1975) Desensitization, behavior rehearsal, self-instructional training and placebo effects on assertive refusal behaviour. *European Journal of Behaviour Analysis Modification,* 1, 30–44.

TROWER, P. E. (1971) A procedure for assessment and modification of behavior in a single case. M.Sc. thesis. Leeds University.

TROWER, P. E., YARDLEY, K. M., BRYANT, B.M. AND SHAW, P. H. (in press) The treatment of social failure: a comparison of anxiety-reduction and skills-acquisition procedures on two social problems. *Behavior Modification.*

ULLRICH DE MUYNCK, R. AND ULLRICH, R. (1972) The efficiency of a standardised assertive training programme. (ATP) Paper presented at Second Conference of European Association for Behaviour Therapy Modification, Wexford, Ireland.

VITALO, R. (1971) Teaching improved interpersonal functioning as a preferred mode of treatment. *Journal of Clinical Psychology*, 22, 166–71.

WOLPE, J. (1958) *Psychotherapy by Reciprocal Inhibition*. Stanford, Calif.: University Press.

WOLPE, J. (1970) The instigation of assertive behavior: Transcripts from two cases. *Journal of Behavior Therapy and Experimental Psychiatry*, 1, 145–51.

WOLPE, J. (1973a) *The Practice of Behaviour Therapy*. Oxford: Pergamon.

WOLPE, J. (1973b) Supervision Transcript V: Mainly about assertive training. *Behavior Therapy*, 4, 141–8.

YARDLEY, K. M. (1976) Training in feminine skills in a male transsexual: a pre-operative procedure. *British Journal of Medical Psychology*, 49, 329–39.

YOUNG, E. R., RIMM, D. C. AND KENNEDY, T. D. (1973) An experimental investigation of modeling and verbal reinforcement in the modification of assertive behaviour. *Behaviour Research and Therapy*, 11, 317–19.

Part Two

6   Assessment

Information is needed both for selecting suitable patients and for planning training programmes. Much of the information required is of a rather different kind from that usually obtained in clinical assessment, and falls into three main areas.

1. Past and current relationships. This area is concerned with difficulties experienced with various kinds of people in various settings, and which are of an enduring nature and not merely the temporary result of, for example, being depressed.

2. Social situations. This deals with difficulties complained of in specific social situations.

3. Behaviour. This refers to inadequate social performance shown in social situations.

Information of the first and second kind is obtained mainly in interview, and the third from direct observation. In the procedure described below we assume that the assessor has established that the patient has a social problem rather than one, for instance, of organic origin.

PAST AND CURRENT RELATIONSHIPS AND ACTIVITIES

Some of the information obtained in a traditional psychiatric interview will be of relevance, but the emphasis should be on the patient's past and current social relationships and activities rather than his symptoms and diagnosis.

(a) Prominence should be given to what clinicians call 'premorbid personality' – on whether the patient was a good mixer in childhood and adolescence and earlier adulthood. This information is related to social inadequacy (see chapter 3). Questions should deal with the number, type and closeness of friends, the number of dates and the success of heterosexual (and other sexual) relationships, the extent and nature of social activities, and the motivation to seek friends rather than solitude. A description of the personalities of parents and siblings and the patient's early relationship with them is also useful in producing clues to current social difficulties.

(b) The assessment should also explore the current social situation, such as whether the patient is living at home, in digs, and so on; the people who are currently influencing his social life; the amount of social contact he has at home, work and elsewhere, and with family, relatives, friends and acquaintances.

Information should be collected both from the patient and from a relative, if possible. We find it useful to summarise this information in a form such as suggested on p. 138.

DIFFICULTY IN SOCIAL SITUATIONS

The purpose of this part of the assessment is to find out (i) what situations the patient finds most difficult and (ii) in terms of the social skills model, the specific nature of his difficulty, for example whether it was due to faulty perception, poor performance and so on. Information in this area should be detailed and specific, concentrating on particular occasions, establishing what actually happened, and the precise feelings of discomfort.

(a) The patient should first be asked generally what situations he finds difficult. This provides him with the opportunity to get off his chest the problems he most wants to talk about. We have found it useful to pinpoint a specific occasion for discussion, preferably the last time he found himself in this situation, as he should have greater ease in recalling what happened and what went wrong that time. The next stage is to go systematically through a list of situations, and our Social Situations Questionnaire (pp. 139–43) is intended for this purpose. The patient completes this questionnaire, which asks both for the degree of difficulty felt and how frequently the situation is encountered.

(b) The therapist explores the nature of the difficulties in those situations for which the patient reported moderate difficulty or worse. This can be achieved by first getting the patient to report, in detail, the last situation of this kind that he remembers, and then questioning him on various aspects of his performance (see p. 144). In cases of difficulty, the following additional questions are often useful in getting information on various levels of failure:

Goals. What were the patient's motives in this situation? Does he have a clear idea of what he wants, e.g. dating a girl, being accepted etc.? If he denies having goals, is he blocking them out, due perhaps to anxiety or a history of failure? Or is he seeking 'sick' goals as compensation for real ones, for similar reasons?

Planning. Does he have a good idea of what the problem is? Does he have any plans or strategies for coping with the problem situations? Does he fail to consider alternative responses, or does he seem unable to use these alternatives?

Perception. How does the patient interpret this situation? Does his interpretation seem distorted, perhaps by fear of negative evaluation or paranoia? Is he blocking out feedback from others? Or if his interpretations are accurate, is the feedback punishing or unrealistic? If punishing, is this because his behaviour is producing a negative effect in others?

Performance. Is his performance inadequate, and does he know this? Is the poor performance due to temporary anxiety or depression, or a history of poor socialisation? Is his difficulty generalised or specific to certain situations?

BEHAVIOUR

The aim of this part of the assessment is to establish both whether the patient lacks behavioural skills in normal social encounters and also which particular skills are deficient.

To do this, it is necessary (a) to observe the patient's social performance and (b) to make records and ratings from these observations.

(a) For obvious reasons, typical social behaviour cannot be sampled in a clinical interview and, ideally, observations of the patient should be obtained from people in different situations – e.g. from relatives, friends, nurses, therapists, in such situations as at home, in the street, at work, in the hospital. However, in practice we usually have to settle for a smaller sample, and one way is to get the patient to participate in a simulated social situation. The Social Interaction Test (page 144) is a simulation which we have developed out of eight years of trial and error experience of assessing several hundred patients. It samples a range of different skills, such as listening, speaking, handling silences and coping with a difficult person. Despite being structured and standardised, patients report that the test situation is realistic. Therapists may try less structured encounters but may find their ratings to be less reliable and the information obtained less comprehensive.

However, the S.I.T. only samples one kind of situation – talking to strangers – and therapists should supplement this by interviewing informants who have outside contact with the patients.

(b) The rating scale* (page 145) is designed to help judges record their observations systematically, both at a behavioural and a more general level, and to help ensure that disagreements are not due to errors. We have found that genuine disagreements provide useful information and should not be discounted as error variance.

The systematic observation of behaviour is itself a skill which therapists can acquire through practice – and indeed we recommend extensive practice in using the rating scale provided.

SUMMARY

The information obtained in assessment can now be summarised to help to tailor a treatment programme to an individual. In organising a programme for a group, it may be necessary to include some aspects which are important for some individuals but redundant for others, but often this compromise is no bad thing, producing some unexpected advantages. Some suggestions on the 'mix' of groups are given in the manual (page 177). Below, we give two simplified examples of how the assessment can be used to help in training, the first for general social inadequacy, the other for specific phobia. As these show, we recommend therapists to draw on other treatments where necessary, such as drugs, psychotherapy and anxiety-reducing behaviour therapies.

* A paper on reliability and validity of the scale is in preparation.

Summary of difficulties	Skills problem	Training and other treatment
(a) General problem of getting on with peers, particularly socially and at work, and with girls.	*Goals* Denies having any social goals, probably due to depression and history of failure.	Clarification of goals. Psychotherapy? Antidepressants?
	Perception Blocking out, probably due to fear of negative evaluation	Observation and gaze training in groups. Systematic desensitisation.
	Performance Unrewarding Unassertive	Basic training in speaking, listening, meshing and social routines. Situation training for peer encounters.
	Planning Fails to consider and implement alternatives.	Tactics and strategies training.
(b) Specific fear of vomiting in public, leading to avoidance of social and business encounters.	*Goals* No problem	—
	Perception No problem	—
	Performance Failure to cope with invitations and eating out, due to anxiety	Training in apologies, accounts and refusals and other relevant routines. Behaviour rehearsal and in vivo practice of eating out. Systematic desensitisation. Anxiolytic drugs?
	Planning Cannot implement alternatives.	Situation-specific training in tactics and strategies.

Assessment Measures

Relationships

NAME:

DATE:

RELATIONSHIPS

Mixing with others	*Childhood*	*Adolescence*	*Since Adolescence*
1. Had many friends and mixed easily	. . . . .	. . . . .	. . . . .
2. Mixed only with close friend or group of friends	. . . . .	. . . . .	. . . . .
3. No close friends; very few friends, never quite accepted by friends	. . . . .	. . . . .	. . . . .
4. Quiet; aloof; preferred to be by self	. . . . .	. . . . .	. . . . .
5. Antisocial	. . . . .	. . . . .	. . . . .

*Interest in opposite sex**

1. Shows healthy interest in opposite sex with regular 'dating' or marriage	. . . . .	. . . . .
2. Some interest; circle of friends included opposite sex; some attempts at 'dating'	. . . . .	. . . . .
3. Little interest in opposite sex; unsuccessful encounters with them; preferred to be with own sex	. . . . .	. . . . .
4. Little interest in opposite or same sex; preferred to be by self	. . . . .	. . . . .
5. Definitely avoided by opposite sex	. . . . .	. . . . .

*Scale can be modified for homosexual clients.

Social Situations Questionnaire

This questionnaire is concerned with how people get on in social situations, that is, situations involving being with other people, talking to them etc.

PAGE ONE: HOW DIFFICULT?

The first page deals with how much difficulty, if any, *you* have in these situations. Having difficulty means that the situation makes you feel ANXIOUS or UNCOMFORTABLE, either because you don't know what to do, or because you feel frightened, embarrassed or self-conscious.

1. Across the top of page 1 you will see five different choices of difficulty, each with a number underneath (e.g. 'no difficulty' =0).
2. Down the left hand side of the page are listed 30 situations you might encounter which some people have said they find difficult. If some of these situations are ones in which you have never found yourself, please imagine how you would feel if you did.
3. Down the right hand side of the page are two columns which refer to two different points in time. They are headed (a) the present time; (b) this time a year ago.

For each situation, and for each point in time, select the choice of difficulty which most closely fits how you feel, and write the number of your choice in the appropriate column.

Examples

	Present time	Year ago
A. Going to a public meeting	..3..	..1..
B. Going to the cinema	..0..	..0..

Example A means that someone had great difficulty (3) at the present time, and slight difficulty (1) a year ago.

Example B means that someone had no difficulty (0) at either of these points in time.

Please note : Choice 'avoidance if possible' should only be used if you find the situation so difficult that you would avoid it whenever you could. It should NOT be used for situations you avoid because they are not to your taste – e.g. not going to concerts because you dislike music.

140   Social skills and mental health

The second page deals with how often you have found yourself in each of the 22 situations listed on the left hand side of the page. The procedure is exactly the same as that for page 1.

1. Across the top of page 2 are seven different 'how often' choices, each with a number underneath it (e.g. 'at least once a week' =2).
2. Down the right hand side of the page are two columns referring to two three-month periods: (a) the last three months · and (b) the same three months a year ago.

For each situation, and for each three month period, select a 'how often' choice and write the number in the appropriate column.

Please note : Choice 'never' (7) means that you have never in your life been in that particular situation. It should therefore be used in both columns.

PAGE ONE

Date: Sex: Name: . . . .

No difficulty 0	Slight difficulty 1	Moderate difficulty 2	Great difficulty 3	Avoidance if possible 4
			At the present time	This time a year ago

1. Walking down the street . . . .   ———   ———
2. Going into shops . . . .   ———   ———
3. Going on public transport . . . .   ———   ———
4. Going into pubs . . . .   ———   ———
5. Going to parties . . . .   ———   ———
6. Mixing with people at work . . . .   ———   ———
7. Making friends of your own age . . . .   ———   ———
8. Going out with someone you are
   sexually attracted to . . . .   ———   ———
9. Being with a group of the same sex and
   roughly the same age as you . . . .   ———   ———
10. Being with a group containing both men
    and women of roughly the same age as
    you . . . .   ———   ———
11. Being with a group of the opposite sex of
    roughly the same age as you . . . .   ———   ———
12. Entertaining people in your home,
    lodgings etc. . . . .   ———   ———
13. Going into restaurants or cafes . . . .   ———   ———
14. Going to dances, dance halls or
    discotheques . . . .   ———   ———
15. Being with older people . . . .   ———   ———
16. Being with younger people . . . .   ———   ———
17. Going into a room full of people . . . .   ———   ———
18. Meeting strangers . . . .   ———   ———
19. Being with people you don't know very well   ———   ———
20. Being with friends . . . .   ———   ———

21. Approaching others – making the first move in starting up a friendship . . . .   ———   ———

22. Making ordinary decisions affecting others (e.g. what to do together in the evening) .   ———   ———

23. Being with only one other person rather than a group . . . .   ———   ———

24. Getting to know people in depth . . . .   ———   ———

25. Taking the initiative in keeping a conversation going . . . .   ———   ———

26. Looking at people directly in the eyes . . .   ———   ———

27. Disagreeing with what other people are saying and putting forward your own views   ———   ———

28. People standing or sitting very close to you   ———   ———

29. Talking about yourself and your feelings in a conversation . . . .   ———   ———

30. People looking at you . . . .   ———   ———

PAGE TWO

Every day or almost every day 1	At least once a week 2	At least once a fortnight 3	At least once a month 4	Once or twice in three months 5	Not at all in three months 6	Never 7
				Last three months ———	Three month period a year ago ———	

1. Walking down the street . . . .   ———   ———

2. Going to the shops . . . .   ———   ———

3. Going on public transport . . . .   ———   ———

4. Going into pubs . . . .   ———   ———

5. Going to parties . . . .   ———   ———

6. Mixing with people at work . . . .   ———   ———

7. Making friends of your own age ....   ——————   ——————

8. Going out with someone you are
   sexually attracted to ....   ——————   ——————

9. Being with a group of the same sex and
   roughly the same age as you ....   ——————   ——————

10. Being with a group containing both men
    and women of roughly the same age as
    you ....   ——————   ——————

11. Being with a group of the opposite sex
    of roughly the same age as you ....   ——————   ——————

12. Entertaining people in your home,
    lodgings, etc. ....   ——————   ——————

13. Going into restaurants or cafes ....   ——————   ——————

14. Going to dances, dance halls or
    discotheques ....   ——————   ——————

15. Being with older people ....   ——————   ——————

16. Being with younger people ....   ——————   ——————

17. Going into a room full of people ......   ——————   ——————

18. Meeting strangers ....   ——————   ——————

19. Being with people you don't know very
    well ....   ——————   ——————

20. Being with friends ....   ——————   ——————

21. Approaching others – making the first
    move in starting up a friendship ....   ——————   ——————

22. Making ordinary decisions affecting
    others (e.g. what to do together in the
    evening) ....   ——————   ——————

Comments If you wish to add any comments about your ratings of difficulty
or frequency, please do so below and continue overleaf if necessary.

Social situations interview

The therapist can use the following questions to probe into the nature of the social difficulties reported in the Social Situations Questionnaire. The therapist should take each situation in turn which is rated 2, 3 or 4 (moderate or great difficulty, or avoidance).

What was the situation?

When and where did it happen?

Who was involved?

What led up to this?

What did you want to do in this situation?

What actually happened?

What did you feel?

What did you think of the others?

Social interaction test

Patients are told that it is essential for training purposes that we observe their actual performance in a situation they might encounter in everyday life. The situation we have chosen resembles a casual three-person encounter between strangers, such as might occur at a social club. The patients are told that the two strangers they will meet are just ordinary people (in our case a woman secretary and a male student), who are in no way connected with their treatment and who think that this encounter is part of a social psychology experiment. We stress that this is not an interview and they should not talk about their problems as they would to the doctor. They are assured that the filming (if any) and the whole procedure are entirely confidential.

The test takes place in a room set up as a lounge, preferably equipped with video apparatus. The patient and confederates are introduced and shown to their seats, with the following instructions: 'As you all know, this is part of an experiment in communication, so I wonder if you (patient) would start the ball rolling by talking about yourself, what you do, where you come from, and so on, and then keep the conversation going for four minutes (indicate the clock), and then would you (woman confederate) do the same for the next four minutes? It is not meant to be a speech – the idea is simply to give one person the responsibility for keeping the conversation going, and then another person – so you can talk or ask questions or carry on any kind of conversation you want. Finally, would you (male confederate) chip in whenever you feel like it?'

Unknown to the patient, some of the confederates' behaviour is prepared. The woman adopts a warm and friendly style. She uses full listener responses while the patient talks, with helpful non-directive questions where necessary, but interrupts this with at least one period of non-response. She also interrupts her own period of talking with a similar period of non-response. The non-response periods should last about 15 seconds. The male confederate adopts a cold and dominant style. After 8 minutes he takes over control of the conversation by asking the patient questions about his work, interests, etc., but withholds any positive feedback and discloses little information about himself. The confederates should not be therapists and should preferably come from a similar social class to the patient's. They should have no other involvement with the patient, either prior to or following the test.

Rating scale

The scale is in two parts. The first part deals with specific elements – verbal and non-verbal behaviour and physical appearance – and the second with psychological impressions, such as warmth and dominance, which are formed from these elements.

The rater proceeds by first concentrating on the patient's *actual behaviour*, scoring the elements as he goes along, in the way described in the scale (pp. 146–56).

After completing the elements section, the rater then concentrates on the *general impression* the patient gives, and notes down his impressions on thirteen seven-point, bipolar adjective scales (p. 156).

Finally, the rater draws together the two aspects of the rating scale by writing behavioural descriptions for some of the general impressions he considers most faulty. Two examples of this are given in the companion rating guide (pp. 167–8).

Raters should watch the film of the interaction test through once, and then work systematically through the scale while watching further replays. If no video is available ratings can be made immediately after the interaction, with the aid of a tape recording.

The raters should include the two confederates from the inter-action test, and at least one of the therapists. All raters should familiarise themselves with the scale and the definitions of the elements, through the companion rating guide, and rate some sample films before rating the patient. There will usually be reasonable agreement on the elements and adjectives which most characterise the deficits.

In making their judgments, raters should bear the following points in mind:

(a) The appropriateness of the behaviour should be thought of in the context of the situation being observed. Thus, for example, intimate behaviour which might be acceptable at a party, would not be appropriate in the interaction test.

(b) Raters should also be cautious about making generalisa-tions from behaviour in the observed situation to others. Recent evidence (Rutter 1975) suggests that patients' behaviour is more dependent on specific situations than previously realised.

(c) The ratings should be thought of in relation to normal social behaviour and not psychiatric disorders. Thus, for example, while gaze avoidance might be appropriate to a depressed state in a clinical interview, it would be inappropriate in normal social interaction.

(d) Related to the above, the therapist should supplement his observations from the interaction test with observations made in other settings (interview, reports by others), and adjust his ratings where necessary. Some parts of the scale cannot in any case be rated from the interaction test, and information must be obtained elsewhere.

VOICE QUALITY

1. *Volume*

0   Normal volume
1(a) Quiet but can be heard without difficulty
 (b) Rather loud but not unpleasant
2(a) Too quiet and difficult to hear
 (b) Too loud and rather unpleasant
3(a) Abnormally quiet and often inaudible
 (b) Abnormally loud and unpleasant

4(a) Inaudible
 (b) Extremely loud (shouting)

2. *Tone*

0   Normal voice quality

1   Fair voice quality – not unpleasant or boring

2   Unmodulated and poor voice quality (dull, flat, thin, etc.). Rather unpleasant and boring

3   Abnormally unmodulated and expressionless. Unpleasant and boring.

4   Extremely flat, expressionless and poor quality. Very unpleasant and boring.

3. *Pitch*

0   Normal pitch

1   Moderately high or low or monotonous but not unpleasant

2   Too high or low or monotonous and rather unpleasant

3   Abnormally high, low or monotonous and unpleasant

4   Extremely high, low or monotonous and unpleasant

4. *Clarity*

0   Normal clarity

1(a) Tends to mumble, slur or drawl words but not unclear
 (b) Tends to clip, over-articulate words but not unpleasant

2(a) Too much mumbling, slurring and drawling. Difficult to understand
 (b) Too much clipping, over-articulation. Rather unpleasant

3(a) Abnormally unclear enunciation. Often impossible to understand
 (b) Abnormally precise and over-articulated. Unpleasant

4(a) Extremely unclear. Impossible to understand.
 (b) Extremely over-articulated. Very unpleasant.

5. *Pace*

0   Normal Pace

1(a) Slow but not difficult to follow
 (b) Fast but not difficult to follow

2(a) Too slow and difficult to follow
 (b) Too fast and difficult to follow

3(a) Abnormally slow and often impossible to follow
 (b) Abnormally fast and often impossible to follow

4(a) Extremely slow, impossible to follow
 (b) Extremely fast, impossible to follow

6. *Speech disturbances*   0   None

1(a) Occasional stuttering, repetitions, omissions, etc., but no negative impression
 (b) Occasional use of pause fillers but no negative impression

2(a) Too much stuttering, repetition, omission, etc. Negative impression
 (b) Too many pause fillers. Negative impression

3(a) Abnormal stuttering, repetition, omission, etc. Embarrassing
 (b) Abnormally frequent pause fillers. Unpleasant

4(a) Extreme stuttering, repetition, omission etc. Extremely embarrassing
 (b) Extremely frequent pause fillers. Very unpleasant

NON-VERBAL

7. *Proximity*   0   Normal casual/personal range

1(a) Rather distant but no negative impression
 (b) Rather too close but no negative impression

2(a) Too distant. Negative impression
 (b) Too close. Negative impression

3(a) Abnormally distant for casual/personal interaction. Unrewarding
 (b) Abnormally close for casual/personal interaction. Unpleasant

4(a) Outside range for social interaction
 (b) Extremely close and intimate. Very unpleasant

8. *Orientation*

0   Normal orientation for casual/personal interaction

1   Turned slightly away but no negative impression

2   Turned too far away. Negative impression

3   Abnormal orientation – 90 degree angle

4   Turned completely away – more than 90 degree angle. Very unpleasant

9. *Appearance*

0   Normal appearance

1   Unusual appearance but no negative impression

2   Appearance unusual, unattractive, unacceptable. Negative impression

3   Appearance abnormally unusual, unattractive, unacceptable. Unpleasant

4   Appearance extremely unusual, unattractive, unacceptable. Very unpleasant

10. *Face*

0   Normal range of emotional expressions

1(a) Face tends to be inexpressive but not unpleasant

(b) Some mildly negative expressions but not unpleasant

2(a) Face often blank, expressions weak or limited in range. Rather unpleasant

(b) Frequent mildly negative expressions. Rather unpleasant

3(a) Face abnormally blank and range limited. Unpleasant

(b) Some abnormally strong negative expressions. Unpleasant

4(a) Totally blank face. Very unpleasant

(b) Frequent strongly negative expressions. Very unpleasant

11. *Gaze*

0   Normal gaze frequency and pattern

1(a) Tends to avoid looking, but no negative impression

(b) Tends to look too much, but no negative impression

2(a) Looks too little. Negative impression
 (b) Looks too much. Negative impression

3(a) Abnormally infrequent looking. Unrewarding
 (b) Abnormally frequent looking. Unpleasant

4(a) Completely avoids looking. Very unrewarding
 (b) Stares continually. Very unpleasant

12. *Posture tonus*

0   Normal relaxed tonus

1(a) Rather stiff and immobile but no negative impression
 (b) Relaxed and rather slouched but no negative impression

2(a) Too stiff, immobile, symmetrical. Negative impression
 (b) Too relaxed, slouched. Negative impression

3(a) Abnormally stiff, immobile, symmetrical. Unpleasant
 (b) Abnormally slouched. Unpleasant

4(a) Extremely rigid, immobile, symmetrical. Very unpleasant
 (b) Extremely slouched. Very unpleasant

13. *Posture position*

0   Normal open style

1   Slightly reclined or closed but no negative impression

2   Too reclined or closed. Negative impression

3   Abnormally reclined or closed. Unpleasant

4   Extremely reclined, tightly closed. Very unpleasant

14. *Gesture*

0   Normal amount and variety of gesture

1   Limited use of gesture but no negative impression

2   Use of gesture too limited in frequency and range. Negative impression

3   Abnormally limited use of gesture in frequency and range. Unrewarding

4   Never gestures. Very unrewarding

15. *Autistic gesture*

0   Unnoticeable amount of autistic gesture

1   Noticeable level of autistic gesture but no negative impression

2   Too many autistic gestures. Negative impression

3   Abnormal amount of autistic gesture. Embarrassing, stressful

4   Extremely frequent autistic gestures. Extremely embarrassing, stressful.

CONVERSATION

16. *Length*
Note: Rate actual speech, excluding pauses

0   Normal speech length

1(a) Speech brief but no unfavourable impression

(b) Speaks at length but no unfavourable impression

2(a) Speaks too briefly. Negative impression

(b) Speaks too long. Negative impression

3(a) Abnormally brief speech. Unpleasant impression

(b) Abnormally lengthy speech. Unpleasant impression

4(a) Speech monosyllabic. Extremely unpleasant

(b) Speaks at great length. Extremely unpleasant

17. *Generality*

0   Normal mixture of general and specific content

1(a) Content mainly general but no unfavourable impression

(b) Content mainly detailed and specialised but no unfavourable impression

2(a) Content too general and uninformative. Negative impression

    (b) Content too detailed and specialised. Negative impression

3(a) Content abnormally generalised. Irritating impression

  (b) Content abnormally detailed and specialised. Irritating impression

4(a) Content at extremely general level. No information. Very irritating

  (b) Content at extremely detailed and specialised level. Extremely irritating

18. *Formality*	0	Normal level of informal talk
	1(a)	Content rather formal but not uninteresting
	(b)	Content rather personal but no negative impression
	2(a)	Content too formal and uninteresting
	(b)	Content too intimate etc. Negative impression
	3(a)	Content abnormally formal and boring
	(b)	Content abnormally intimate etc. Embarrassing, annoying, etc.
	4(a)	Content extremely formal and boring
	(b)	Content extremely intimate etc. Extremely embarrassing, annoying
19. *Variety*	0	Normal variety of topic
	1	Variety of content lacking but not uninteresting
	2	Too little variety of content. Uninteresting
	3	Abnormally unvaried topic content. Boring
	4	Content all of one kind. Very boring
20. *Humour*	0	Normal level of humour
	1	Little humour but no negative impression
	2	Content too serious – hardly any humour. Negative impression
	3	Content abnormally serious – no humour. Unrewarding
	4	Content extremely serious and humourless. Very unrewarding

21. *Non-verbal*   0   Normal non-verbal accompaniments of
     'grammar'   speech

1   Tends to under-use non-verbal accompaniments of speech but no negative impression

2   Under-uses non-verbal accompaniments of speech. Somewhat confusing, boring

3   Abnormal under-use of non-verbal accompaniments of speech. Confusing, boring

4   Hardly uses any non-verbal accompaniments of speech. Incomprehensible, boring

22. *Feedback*   0   Normal listener feedback

1(a)   Feedback infrequent or some elements omitted but not unpleasant

(b)   Feedback mildy critical or inaccurate but not unpleasant

2(a)   Feedback too infrequent, unvaried. Rather unpleasant

(b)   Feedback too critical or inaccurate. Rather unpleasant

3(a)   Feedback abnormally infrequent, unvaried. Unpleasant

(b)   Feedback abnormally critical, inaccurate. Unpleasant

4(a)   No feedback. Very unpleasant

(b)   Very critical or inaccurate feedback. Very unpleasant

23. *Meshing*   0   Normal meshing

1(a)   Responses delayed but no negative impression

(b)   Interrupts occasionally but no negative impression

2(a)   Responses too delayed. Negative impression

(b)   Rather too many interruptions, negative impression

3(a) Responses abnormally delayed. Unpleasant
 (b) Abnormally frequent or long interruptions. Annoying

4(a) Responses extremely delayed. Very unpleasant
 (b) Interruptions extremely frequent or long. Very annoying

24. *Turn taking*

0 Normal turn taking
1(a) Tends to offer or take up floor infrequently, but no negative impression
 (b) Offers or takes up floor frequently but no negative impression

2(a) Offers or spontaneously takes up floor too infrequently. Negative impression.
 (b) Offers or takes up floor too frequently. Negative impression

3(a) Abnormally infrequent offering or spontaneous taking up floor. Unrewarding
 (b) Abnormally frequent offering or taking up floor. Irritating

4(a) Never offers or spontaneously takes up floor. Very unrewarding
 (b) Continually offers or takes up floor. Very irritating

25. *Questions*

0 Normal use of varied questions
1(a) Few or unvaried questions but no negative impression
 (b) Frequent use of questions but no negative impression

2(a) Questions too few and unvaried. Negative impression
 (b) Questions too frequent. Negative impression

3(a) Abnormally infrequent or unvaried questions. Unrewarding
 (b) Abnormally frequent questions. Unpleasant

4(a) Never asks questions. Very unrewarding
 (b) Continually asks questions. Very unpleasant

26. *Supportive routines*   0   Normal use of main routines

1   Low use of routines but no negative impression

2   Important routines performed too infrequently and inadequately. Negative impression

3   Important routines omitted. Unpleasant

4   Essential routines omitted. Very unpleasant

27. *Assertive routines*   0   Normal use of main assertive routines

1(a) Low use of assertive routines but no negative impression
 (b) High use of assertive routines but no negative impression

2(a) Assertive routines performed too infrequently or inadequately. Negative impression
 (b) Assertive routines performed too frequently. Negative impression

3(a) Important assertive routines omitted. Abnormally submissive impression
 (b) Abnormally frequent use of assertive routines. Unpleasant

4(a) Essential assertive routines omitted. Extremely submissive impression
 (b) Continuous use of assertive routines. Very unpleasant

28. *Behaviour in public*   0   Normal prescribed behaviour

1   Some minor transgression of publicly prescribed behaviour but no negative impression

2   Frequent minor transgression of public behaviour

3   Some major transgressions of public behaviour. Unpleasant

4   Frequent major transgressions of public behaviour. Very unpleasant

29. *Situation-specific routines*	0	Normal prescribed behaviour
	1	Some minor transgressions of situation rules but no negative impression
	2	Frequent minor transgression of situation rules. Negative impression
	3	Some major transgression of situation rules. Unpleasant
	4	Frequent major transgressions of situation rules.

GENERAL IMPRESSIONS

Warm/like	—	—	—	—	—	—	— Cold/dislike
Superior/dominant	—	—	—	—	—	—	— Inferior/submissive
Socially anxious	—	—	—	—	—	—	— Relaxed
Happy	—	—	—	—	—	—	— Sad
Rewarding	—	—	—	—	—	—	— Unrewarding
Controlling	—	—	—	—	—	—	— Uncontrolling
Feminine	—	—	—	—	—	—	— Masculine
Attractive	—	—	—	—	—	—	— Unattractive
Poised	—	—	—	—	—	—	— Awkward
Passive	—	—	—	—	—	—	— Active
Difficult	—	—	—	—	—	—	— Easy
Emotional	—	—	—	—	—	—	— Unemotional
Socially skilled	—	—	—	—	—	—	— Socially unskilled

Behavioural description (1):

Behavioural description (2):

Rating guide

This guide gives a brief description and explanation of the elements in the rating scale (except where more detail is given elsewhere), and is designed to help sharpen the raters' observation skills and increase agreement on scores. In addition, the guide is offered as a referral source for use throughout training, to help pick out the more subtle deficiencies which may need special attention. There is more information of this kind in chapter 2.

VOICE QUALITY

There are three important aspects of vocalisation. First, sound as a basic medium of communication; second, sound as a communicator of feelings, attitudes and personality; and third, sound which gives emphasis and meaning to speech.

1. *Volume.* The most basic function of volume is to carry a message to a potential listener, and the obvious – and common – deficit is a volume level too low to serve this function, leading e.g. to the speaker being ignored or the listener irritated. In addition, variations in the sound amplitude carry the following meanings: Very soft = sadness, affection, submissiveness; moderate = pleasantness, activity, happiness; loud = dominance, confidence, extraversion, persuasiveness. Finally, the 'prosodic' rules of patterns of loudness govern the meaning and emphasis given to words. Incorrect use of loudness patterns can confuse the message and produce dull speech.

2. *Tone.* Tone is the vocal quality or resonance of the voice produced mainly as a result of the shape of the oral cavities. Tonal variations are numerous, e.g. dull, flat, thin, blaring, resonant, etc. Voice quality has an aesthetic aspect, resonant tone being the most attractive, thin, nasal, raucous etc. being unattractive. Tonal variations carry a number of positive meanings, e.g. resonance = sadness, dominance, affection; throaty = older, realistic, mature, sophisticated, well adjusted. Negative tones, some common among patients, are: sharp voice = complaining, helpless; flat voice = flabby, sickly, depressed; hollow voice = debilitated, weak; breathy voice = anxious; thin voice = submissiveness.

3. *Pitch.* Pitch is the vocal note, which, like the sound amplitude of volume, varies along a continuum from high to low sound frequency. The best known differences in range are between male and female, and one form of deficit is a pitch level outside the patient's gender range. Some commonly found meanings are: High pitch with soft volume = submissiveness, grief; with loud volume = activity, potency, anger; with variable volume = fear,

surprise, grief. Low pitch with loud volume = dominance; with variable volume = pleasantness; with soft volume = boredom, sadness. High variation = feminine, dynamic, aesthetically inclined, pleasant, active, happy, surprised; low variation = depressed, disinterested; rising pitch = cheerful; falling pitch = depressed. Pitch variation also gives meaning, colour and emphasis to speech.

4. *Clarity*.   Clarity ranges from extreme drawl to extreme clipping. This continuum is concerned both with the basic comprehensibility of communication, and with meaning and accent. The meanings of clarity include the following: Clipped = upper social class, anger, impatience; slurred = lower social class, sadness, affection, boredom.

5. *Pace*.   As with clarity, pace varies on a continuum concerned both with basic comprehensibility at the extremes, and with psychological and linguistic meaning. Psychological meanings include: Fast = pleasantness, activity, potency, anger, anxiety, happiness, surprise, persuasiveness, assertiveness, 'high achievement', animation, extraversion; slow = sadness, affection, boredom, disgust. In speech, pacing functions like punctuation in written English, e.g. pauses at grammatical junctures.

6. *Speech disturbances*.   Speech disturbances are traditionally divided into two main kinds: 'ums' and 'ers' which speakers use to fill pauses and which represent 'thinking time', and the so-called 'non-ah' disturbances which are signs of anxiety and include sentence changes, repetitions, stuttering, omissions (leaving out a word or leaving it unfinished), sentence incompletion, tongue slips and nonsense sounds. Excessive use of pause fillers may be interpreted as boredom, and excessive unfilled pauses may be interpreted as anger or contempt, though both extremes could suggest anxiety.

NON-VERBAL

7. *Proximity*.   The meaning of distance between two people can be described in terms of an intimacy-formality dimension, and has been divided up interaction zones in the following way:

intimate – 18 inches; personal, 18 inches to 4 feet; social-consultative – 9 to 12 feet; public, 12 feet and above. These conventional boundaries may be broken inappropriately without a proper change in the relationship; or the individual may communicate unintended coldness and dislike by taking up a distant position.

8. *Orientation.* Degrees of orientation signal degrees of intimacy/formality in much the same way as proximity – the more face-to-face the orientation, the more intimate the relationship, and vice versa. Deficits would therefore be similar, e.g. orienting away and communicating coldness in a personal encounter.

9. *Physical appearance.* Physical appearance has numerous effects on social interaction, and poor management in appearance can lead to negative behaviour and impressions, particularly in certain situations, such as interviews, parties and dating, visiting, theatre-going, etc., i.e. where the presentation of self is important. The main elements of physical appearance and the important information conveyed include the following:

Elements

Face (thickness of lips, height of forehead, deep/shallow set eyes, etc.)

Clothes (colour, style, quality)

Hair (colour, style, length)

Decoration (rings, badges, jewellery)

Skin (complexion, colour, lines, wrinkles)

Cosmetics (make-up, scent, after-shave, etc.)

Beard and moustache (colour, style, length)

Accessories (spectacles, cigarettes, pipe, gloves, hat etc.)

Physique (height, fatness, muscularity, figure, deformity)

Neatness (hair in place, shaven, etc.)

Cleanliness (hair, finger nails, etc.)

Impressions

Age
Gender identity
Sexuality
Attractiveness
Social class
Status
Conformity
Intelligence
Personality
Emotionality
Fashionability
and taste

10. *Face.*   The face is the most important and most complex area
for non-verbal signalling. We will confine our attention to two
main functions: (a) expression of emotion and attitude, and (b)
accompaniments of speech.

(a) There are six primary expressions of emotions and three main
areas of the face responsible for signalling them (see page 196).
Expression of the primary emotions is said to be innate and
universal (the affect display system) but these are modified by
cultural learning (display rules) in four ways: intensified, de-
intensified, masked or blended, the last of these involving the
display of two emotions at the same time, e.g. felt anger blended
with a social smile.

(b) A rapid sequence of facial movements accompanies, and is
subordinate to, speech and is used by speakers to emphasise, frame
and in other ways elaborate the spoken word, and by listeners to
reflect and comment upon the speaker's utterance.

A great deal more information on the face is given in various
parts of the manual and will not be repeated here.

11. *Gaze.*   Gaze is unique in being both a channel (receiver) and
signal (sender), and one kind of deficiency, gaze avoidance, is thus
doubly serious, being a failure on the one hand to get social
feedback and on the other giving negative impressions such as
dislike, boredom, etc.

Some of the meanings and functions of gaze patterns are:
(a) Attitudes. People who look more are seen as likeable, but
extreme staring is seen as hostile and/or dominant and confident.
Less looking communicates nervousness and lack of confidence.
Certain interaction sequences have yet further meanings, e.g.
breaking gaze first is a signal of submission. Pupil dilation signals
liking and likeability. (b) More looking intensifies the impression
of some emotions, like anger, while less looking intensifies others,
e.g. shame. (c) Speech accompaniment. Gaze is used in conjunction with conversation to synchronise (see *Turn taking*, p. 154),
accompany or comment on the spoken word. People look twice
as much while listening, and while speaking look during grammatical breaks, points of emphasis and ends of utterances.
Generally, more listener looking produces more speaker response,
more speaker looking is seen as more persuasive and confident.

The average amount of time people spend looking, in a two-person social conversation, is as follows:

Individual gaze	60 per cent
while listening	75 per cent
while talking	40 per cent
length of glance	3 seconds
Eye contact (mutual glance)	30 per cent
length of mutual glance	$1\frac{1}{2}$ seconds

There are wide variations due to distance, sex combination and personality.

12. *Posture tonus.* This element is concerned with one aspect of posture – the relaxation/tension of the body musculature and the meanings that variations on this dimension signify. (a) Attitudes. Posture probably encodes interpersonal attitudes more than other non-verbal components. Relaxation of the body is seen as a sign of dominance and is manifested by asymmetrical (sprawled) arm and leg positions, sideways or backwards lean and hand relaxation. Conversely, tense, symmetrical positions suggest submissiveness and anxiety. However, certain kinds of *high* muscular tonus are associated with dominance, and, in men, courtship intentions, namely 'thoracico-lumbar display', i.e. squared shoulders, expanded chest. *Low* tonus – sloping shoulders and neck, deflated chest – is associated with submissiveness and depression. (b) Emotion. Posture tension indicates not so much the content of emotion (this is done more by the face, voice and verbal content) but rather the intensity, increased tension indicating increased emotion. However, there are exceptions (see below), such as depression, indifference and anger.

13. *Posture position.* Various posture positions form an additional communication channel, including the following features. (a) Attitudes. A number of posture positions which reduce the distance and increase the openness to another are warm, friendly, intimate, while the reverse positions are seen as cold, unfriendly etc. The 'warm' positions are forward lean, open arms and legs, arms extended towards other. Other attitude positions include: leaning back, hands clasped at back of head = dominance or surprise; arms coiled, stretching down, head down and to side = shyness; legs apart, arms akimbo, sideways lean = determination. (b) Emotions. Some evidence shows that posture can communicate

specific emotions including: shoulder shrug, arms raised, hands outstretched = indifference; forward lean, arms outstretched, fists clenched = anger. Various kinds of pelvic movement, legs crossing and uncrossing (in women) = flirtation.

(c) Accompaniments of speech. Major posture changes are used to mark off larger units of speech, as in changes of topic, to give emphasis and to signal taking up or handing over the floor. (See *Non-verbal grammar*, p. 153, and *Turn taking*, p. 154).

14. *Gesture.*   There are at least five functions of gesture which are displayed in characteristic behaviour patterns:

Function	*Behaviour*
Emblems	
Illustrators	Hand shapes
Affect displays	Hand, arm and head movements
	Hands together
Regulators	Hands to face or body
Adaptors	

Emblems. There is a group of gestures which have a specific conventional meaning of their own or which can be translated into words, e.g. a hand-shake, fist clench, head nod, clapping, rubbing hands, thumbs down, pat on back, waving.

Illustrators. Hand movements can illustrate speech by pointing, showing a spatial relationship (under, inside), showing a bodily action ('kinetographs'), drawing a picture ('pictographs'), showing a direction of thought ('ideographs'). One of the most common usages in conversation is 'I' and 'You' by small sweeps of the hand, except in conjunction with postures (see previous section).

Affect displays. This group is taken here to mean those gestures which are consciously used to disclose, not conceal, feeling. In fact, gestures are a poor channel of emotion expression. General hand and arm movements signal high arousal and excitement, tensed hands and arms intensify emotion, but little is known about patterns for specific emotions.

Regulators. These are used to manage the synchronising of speech and speaking turns (see *Turn taking*, p. 154), to give emphasis and to mark off clauses of speech (see *NV grammar*, p. 153).

Adaptors. This is dealt with as a separate section below.

15. *Autistic gesture*. We include here those gestures termed 'autistic' or 'adaptive', i.e. directed at the self and often unconscious. Some are simply used to satisfy bodily needs – scratching, rubbing – but others more importantly 'leak' information about feelings which are concealed in the major affect display areas (face, voice). There is a direct relationship between emotions negatively sanctioned by society and their 'leakage' in hands and feet. These probably include: covering the eyes = shame; picking and scratching the face = self-blame; finger horizontally placed under nose = lying; picking clothes, tapping feet, foot kicks = anger; caressing movements, leg displays, leg squeezing = flirtatiousness; wringing hands, picking finger nails, restless movements = anxiety.

CONVERSATION

The conversation elements are ordered as follows: the first deal with speech per se, the next with listening and the last with interaction sequences.

16. *Length*.   It has been found in recent studies that the amount of speech of both patients and non-patients contributed very significantly to an overall impression of social skill, and almost certainly more than any other element taken separately. We found that patients judged as socially competent spoke for more than half the time when asked to talk to a stranger, but patients judged socially inadequate spoke only a third of the time. The difference was even greater in a 'listening' role – competent patients spoke 30 per cent of the time, inadequate patients only 10 per cent. Length of speaking has also been found to be related to rewardingness, assertiveness, ability to cope and level of social anxiety.

17. *Generality*. Speaker disclosure has varying degrees of generality, being too general and therefore too brief and uninformative at one extreme, and detailed and specialised, and therefore too long and uninteresting, at the other, for any given context. Thus, at one extreme, a carpenter may say 'Well, it's a job', and at the other, 'There are X kinds of joints. Let's take the housing joint.' Neither of these extremes may be appropriate in, say, a social conversation with a comparative stranger.

18. *Formality*.   The dimension intimate/formal has various sub-components, which are often interrelated: (a) disclosures of factual information about the self or others of varying degrees of a personal/impersonal nature, e.g. 'my sex life. . .' to 'the weather. . .'; (b) verbal expressions of various strengths of emotion and opinion, e.g. 'I love. . .' to 'I'm interested. . .'; (c) informal talk of a chatty kind, e.g. 'idle gossip', jokes etc. to formal talk using third person pronouns and similar lexical forms such as 'It is pleasurable to occupy oneself in. . .'. It has been found that high personal disclosures elicited more personal disclosures from others, and were liked more than low disclosures.

19. *Variety*.   This section is concerned with variety of topic content and is included on the basis of experience rather than research evidence. Variety does not necessarily imply change of topic but rather variety of types of discourse common in social conversations, including humour (see below), story telling, factual information, expression of opinion, thoughts and beliefs etc.

20. *Humour*.   This section is also included on the basis of experience rather than research. The presence or absence of specific humour, such as the telling of jokes, puns etc., as well as a general 'humorous' tone to the conversation, would be considered relevant.

21. *Non-verbal 'grammar'*.   Non-verbal accompaniments of speech have been considered under the non-verbal section but can be usefully grouped here. We are mainly concerned here with the role of NV accompaniments in punctuating, clarifying and 'colouring' speech. Other aspect of NV accompaniments are dealt with under *Feedback* and *Turn taking*. Firstly, NV elements provide punctuation and display the structure of speech. Speakers pause, change or terminate gestures, change their pitch, timing or loudness, their facial expression, look up etc., at the transition points between one clause or sentence and another. They raise their voice pitch, eyebrows and head in asking a question. Secondly, speakers move their hands or head or change their pitch or loudness to give emphasis; thirdly, all these elements are used to 'frame' their utterances as funny, sarcastic, matter-of-fact, etc. Fourthly, speakers use gesture and bodily movement to

spatially illustrate what they are saying. Lack of NV accompaniments can make speech dull, confusing or even meaningless.

22. *Feedback.*   There are three main kinds of listener feedback: attention or comprehension, reflection on the speaker's utterance and commentary on the speaker's utterance. Each of these – or the lack of it – has an effect on the speaker's output. (a) Attention feedback. The listener signals attention by taking up an appropriate distance, orientation and posture, by looking more than 50 per cent of the time, by nodding, grunting or giving verbal affirmatives. The signals mean: 'I'm listening, understand and approve.' Attention feedback invariably increases the output of the speaker. (b) Reflective feedback. Verbal feedback may take a form such as 'You feel . . . because . . .'. It reflects back, at a shallow or deep level, the significance of the speaker's comment and is seen as empathic and rewarding. (c) The listener may comment on the speaker's utterance verbally, by expressing surprise, amusement and so on, and by non-verbal equivalents. These and other aspects of feedback are dealt with more fully in the manual (*Listener skills*, pp. 200–11).

23. *Meshing.*   Speakers synchronise their periods of talk, but when this fails, two kinds of 'asynchrony' occur – simultaneous talking (interruptions) and latencies (periods of non-response). 'Normal' people negotiate this timing and can tolerate fair degrees of asynchrony, and differ from patients in characteristic ways. For instance, non-psychiatric patients are found to interrupt more than either schizophrenics or depressives. However, excessive interruptions or non-response causes stress and can lead to conversation breakdown.

24. *Turn taking.*   Speakers negotiate their speaking turns by a multichannel system of signals, such as verbal content and syntax, intonation, paralinguistic behaviour and gesture. This information is given in detail in the manual (pp. 224–6). When this system breaks down various kinds of failure can occur, in addition to the asynchronies mentioned above. The two main problems concern taking up or handing over the conversation, either of which may be insufficient or excessive. Related problems are suppressing a turn claim and refusing a turn offer.

25. *Questions*.　Questions and indirect equivalents are essential for getting conversation going, getting information, showing an interest in others and affecting the behaviour of others, and their lack of use can produce deficits in all these areas. Types of questions can be categorised in the following ways (see manual, p. 208): general/specific; open/closed; factual/personal; chained/ unchained.

26. *Supportive routines*.　There are a number of social conventions which are made up of a sequence of verbal and non-verbal acts and which may be called routines, e.g. greetings and partings. These may be divided into two main groups: those concerned with politeness and remedying wrongs, affiliativeness and etiquette, which may be classed under *supportiveness*, and those concerned with asserting rights and changing the behaviour of others and which for convenience may be classed under *initiative and assertiveness* (see below). Many supportive routines are in a sense obligatory or 'prescribed', in that their use is expected, and failure to use them may be seen as giving offence, resulting in stress or breakdown in relationships. Routines differ along a dimension of generality, some, such as greetings, being used in nearly all situations, others only in specific settings such as teaching, interviewing, courting. Details of the structure of supportive routines are given in the manual (pp. 229 ff.). Some of the essential or important ones are: greetings, partings, giving thanks, giving praise, paying compliments, offering sympathy, apologising, excusing, reciprocating (accepting or returning others' greetings, thanks, etc.).

27. *Initiative and assertive routines*.　Some assertion routines are essential in that failure to use them may result in the individual being offended, insulted or in some way abused by others, or in failure to alter an undesirable social situation. Research is only now beginning to unravel the structure of these routines, some of which are: making complaints, requests, demands and criticisms, disagreeing, giving commands and advice, refusing and persuading.

28. *Behaviour in public*.　There are social conventions governing behaviour in public such as walking down the street, standing in

queues etc. where little or no interaction takes place. Failure to follow such rules results in offence, for reasons similar to those referred to above. Conventions of this kind include 'body gloss' (use of cues to display acceptable intentions); contact avoidance (depersonalising behaviour, e.g. when face to face with strangers); respecting boundaries (positioning outside other's personal space).

29. *Situation-specific routines.* The behavioural conventions specific to social situations have been likened to the rules of games and sports, the implication being that breaking the rules results in some kind of penalty, in this case of a social nature. Examples of situations where these rules apply include interviews, formal occasions such as ceremonies and meetings, and courtship. Little research has yet been done on situation rules, and the assessor must rely on local informants for information on patients' rule-breaking behaviour.

GENERAL IMPRESSIONS

Nearly all the elements can be combined to produce higher order impressions which are more complex on the one hand, but more familiar in day-to-day life. Below we give two examples of impressions and the elements comprising them.

Cold/dislike may be expressed *vocally* by dull vocal tone and monotonous high pitch; *non-verbally* by maintaining physical distance, avoiding physical contact, orienting the body and/or head away, by gaze aversion or staring and sullen or blank facial expression with little facial movement, by leaning back when seated with arms and legs crossed, and by general bodily immobility with no change of posture and few or no gestures; *verbally*, by brief speech, general and formal discourse, little use of non-verbal accompaniments, and little variety or humour. Feedback is at a minimum, response latencies are long, and there is poor taking up and handing over of the conversation. The cold person uses few questions, is low on supportive routines and may break public and other situation rules.

Inferior/submissive may be expressed *vocally* by a flat, thin tone, low volume, slurring, by speech error repetitions and 'ums'; *non-verbally* by keeping at a distance, hesitant approach behaviour, low body tonus (head and shoulders slumped, chest deflated) *or* rigid posture with limb symmetry, 'fear' face, autistic gestures such as hand to face or fiddling, gaze directed downwards; *verbally*, by too general *or* specific content, poor taking up of conversation, few questions or few assertive routines. A submissive attitude may produce extreme adherence to public and situation rules, especially avoidance of others, and over-use of supportive routines.

7 Training

Introduction

The training manual draws extensively on research into the elements and processes of social interaction as well as clinical experience. However, as the preceding chapters have shown, the information now available is already vast and still rapidly expanding, and we have had to make inevitable sacrifices to keep the manual to reasonable proportions. In the difficult task of selecting the most relevant material we have included areas which, in general, seemed more fundamental, e.g. we have focussed more on face and voice cues and less on gestures and body movements, and more on basic, social conversation rather than specialised applications, such as interviews, business meetings, teaching, courting, public speaking and so on. This inevitably means we will not have covered some areas of deficiency. Some additional behavioural information is given in a descriptive form in the rating scale, and we suggest therapists use this and other sources listed later as background information for training patients whose particular deficits fall into areas not covered in the manual.

A social skills training programme can be tailored to the individual and organised around his particular social problems, or the programme can be a more or less standard 'package' for which the individual is selected by prior screening. The procedure is rather different in the two cases. In the individualised training each session takes as its theme a problem or goal, for instance situations like being interviewed or interviewing, asking for a date, taking part in a group discussion, asserting oneself, or behaviours like gaze aversion, brief or inappropriate talk, giving no verbal or non-verbal feedback. This can be done individually or in open groups where each patient presents his problem in turn, and training may proceed along the lines suggested later (pp. 178–85). The standard training takes the form of a set course, deals systematically with most of the important basic social skills, one or more of which forms the theme of each session. This can also be done individually or in closed groups. Standard training has certain advantages, for instance it can be very thoroughly planned with audio-visual aids and handouts, and then used again and again with little alteration, thus saving on therapists' time; it is useful for trainee therapists in that it is structured, requires less experience and provides a vehicle for gaining clinical experience. The disadvantage is its insensitivity to individual problems, except where these involve basic skills.

The present manual can be used for individual or standard training, or a combination of the two. The therapist can construct his own programme from sections or subsections and from supplementary information as suggested above, according to patients' needs, though therapists should be cautious about leaving out sections of training. The manual may also be used as a standard training programme where deficits are very generalised and fundamental or where extreme feelings of social anxiety and poor self-esteem are present. Even here the therapist should modify and supplement the manual in the light of clinical experience, to make it more appropriate for his patients.

One of the biggest problems of the manual is that it is in a written, as opposed to audio-visual, form, and much of the intuitive 'feel' for training and many of the non-verbal skills and deficits are hard to explain and difficult to understand. However, we have tried to anticipate some of the problems which therapists will meet, and suggest steps to overcome them.

Another problem is getting patients to role-play and rehearse social tasks, particularly speaking skills, in front of others. After all, this is the kind of difficulty which is often at the root of social failure, and it is naive to suppose that patients will find it any easier to do in a training setting amongst other patients.

First, it is essential to carry out a thorough assessment and briefing, in order to get a clear picture of the problem and to enlighten and reassure the patient about his problem and the training procedure to be used (see Assessment Procedure, pp. 133 ff.).

Secondly, the various anxiety management techniques such as desensitisation, flooding, covert modelling, etc. should be used if necessary.

Thirdly, and most important, the training should be organised in such a way as to ease patients slowly and naturally into unaccustomed forms of behaviour, helping them to generate their own preferred styles and strategies. We have tried to achieve this difficult task by following what we regard as the normal, skilled approach to new situations. This often begins with careful observation of the surroundings, cautious interaction in the role, at first, of a listener, followed by greater participation as speaker, and, as confidence grows, bringing about change in situations and others by assertive and rewarding strategies. This is a 'natural' hierarchy of graded tasks, and we have followed a similar sequence in the manual. Any other sequence may risk increasing patients' self-consciousness in the crucial early stages, as well as providing unrealistic general strategy for 'real' life. From the patients' point of view, they will find the training directs their attention towards other people – their behaviour, feelings and reactions – rather than toward the patient. In practice, this means patients are not asked to change their behaviour per se ('Look more, speak louder') but rather to change the *other's* behaviour by giving different feedback. Thus, rather than 'look more', we would suggest 'get the speaker to talk more by giving attention signals such as looking'.

The manual is divided into eleven sections, each with its own list of references. The first section deals with the preliminaries of social skills training, such as therapist skills, induction of the patient, goal setting, social contracts, composition of groups and training routines including the setting, guidance, demonstration, practice, feedback, rehearsal and homework assignments. Finally, we offer some guidance on difficult cases.

Section 2 is an introductory exercise which involves practising a brief conversation and is designed to break the ice and give a framework for the training which follows.

Section 3 deals with observation skills and includes exercises and guidance in getting information about situations and about other people's feelings and attitudes and causes of other people's behaviour, about self-perception, and recognition of verbal and non-verbal cues.

Section 4 is concerned with listening skills and covers verbal and non-verbal reflections, attention feedback, listener commentary and questions.

Section 5 covers speakers' skills, with guidance on things to talk about, and how to gain experience and knowledge and remember information. It gives specific guidance in types of appropriate self-disclosure, such as the level of specificity, informality and emotional content. Attention is also given to the non-verbal accompaniments of speech.

Section 6 concentrates on meshing skills, including the continuity of conversation themes, the timing of utterances and cues for managing speaking turns.

Section 7 focusses on expression of attitudes, such as warmth and assertiveness.

Section 8 deals with everyday social routines such as greeting and parting, giving compliments, praise and other kinds of support, apologising, excusing and saving face. The section also includes assertive routines, such as insisting on rights, and refusing.

Section 9 deals with cognitive planning – or problem-solving – skills, including choosing alternative responses and deciding on general strategies of behaviour, such as being rewarding, controlling, and presenting the self.

Section 10 gives some general guidance on situation training, such as how to carry out role-play simulations of patients' particular difficulties.

Section 11 is a trainee's handbook, which is a supplement designed to be duplicated and handed out to patients, and includes suggested exercise routines for all the training sections and homework assignments for basic conversation skills.

Sections 1 to 10 take the form of a *briefing* for the therapist, a suggested *presentation* routine for the patients and guidance on exercises for practising skills in the studio or clinic 'workshop'.

1. Preliminaries

We suggest the following preparatory work be done before training is attempted: (a) learn the necessary therapist skills; (b) secure the patient's understanding and acceptance of the social skills model; (c) establish a hierarchy of practical goals; (d) negotiate a 'contract' with the patient to carry out homework assignments and keep a continuous record of these and other activities; and (e) decide on group or individual training.

THERAPIST SKILLS

A good therapeutic relationship is an important prerequisite in social skills training, initially to help the patient understand his problem and accept training, and subsequently to increase the therapist's effectiveness as a model and 'reinforcer'. There is good correlational evidence that the 'core conditions' of psychotherapy, namely warmth, empathy and genuineness, are associated with therapeutic improvement in a wide variety of patients (Shapiro 1969); there are now abundant training schemes and manuals for increasing 'helping skills' based on these conditions, and some of these are reviewed in chapter 4. Although not divided up in the same way, the skills in the present manual may also be used to facilitate effectiveness in training, particularly observation and listening skills, and expression of attitudes – particularly warmth. We suggest potential users form themselves into a training group and work through the manual before training patients, both to improve their own skills and to familiarise themselves with the technique.

INDUCTION

Patients construe their own problems in various ways, such as that they are mentally ill, and have expectations about treatment, such as being given medicine. These beliefs may hinder or jeopardise the success of social skills training (Goldstein 1973). The therapist should help the patient understand the social and behavioural causes of his distress, explain the purpose of training and what is involved during the coming sessions.

Concepts for discussing social behaviour with patients

When giving feedback on a patient's performance, or suggesting alternative forms of behaviour, it is necessary to use a suitable vocabulary of terms to describe the behaviour. Some of these terms are not in everyday use, so it is necessary to some extent to teach the patient a basic vocabulary. This teaching is valuable in itself, since it directs attention to the phenomena of social interaction, and through labelling brings them more under cognitive control. Some experiments on microteaching have found that training in the use of a set of interaction categories improves teaching ability as much as role-playing.

For the range of basic, everyday encounters with which we are most concerned in this book a number of verbal and non-verbal elements need to be discussed at this stage and throughout the training. The *verbal* elements include:

asking and answering questions (e.g. open *v.* closed)

giving and seeking information

giving instruction (e.g. requests *v.* commands)

offering and seeking opinions, suggestions

greeting, bidding farewell

apologising, explaining

telling jokes

agreeing, disagreeing

thanking.

The *non-verbal* elements include:

gaze, mutual gaze, glance

facial expression (seven basic emotional expressions, together with cognitive reactions – surprised, puzzled, etc.)

proximity and orientation

voice quality – pitch, loudness, speed, accent

gestures – e.g. head movements accompanying speech (illustrators), and expressing emotions

posture – relaxed-tense, dominant-submissive

appearance – image conveyed by hair, grooming, clothes.

Many patients present problems involving specific social situations or social skills – parties, teaching, public speaking, committees etc. These may require additional concepts for the special moves or social acts required by these situations. Just as there are special moves in chess, water polo and mountaineering, so there are special moves in particular social situations; there are words and phrases to describe these situations which need to be mastered. For example, at a scientific seminar there are such moves as:

Chairman:	introduces session
	asks people to stop talking
Speaker:	gives part of lecture
	shows slides
	demonstrates apparatus
member of audience:	interrupts, disagrees
	interrupts, asks questions

During buying and selling a different set of concepts are involved:

Customer:	asks to see goods
	enquires price of goods
	objects to goods
	gives money to sales person
Sales person:	passes goods to customer
	praises goods.

GOALS

Training depends on the specification of desired goals which the patient fails to achieve because of inadequate skills. Up to ten desired social goals should be selected from the problem situations described in the Social Situations Interview. The following criteria can be used for selection. First, the therapist must secure the patient's agreement on the relevance of goals to ordinary everyday social interaction. Secondly, these situations should be grouped as far as possible under general titles, e.g. 'keeping conversation going', instead of 'talking for half an hour to my neighbour last Sunday'. Thirdly, these situations should be rated (i) for their importance as desired goals, (ii) for the level of anxiety experienced during, or in anticipation of, them; (iii) for the level of anticipated competence in the situation (see List of Social Goals, p. 183).

A scale ranging from 0 to 10 may be used, where 0 is no importance, no anxiety and no incompetence, and 10 is maximum importance, anxiety and incompetence. Goals with higher ratings will usually be most central to the training plan. The situations should be rated before, after, and at every other training session, to give feedback on progress to both patient and therapist. The goals should be listed in order, not of difficulty, but of generality, since training will proceed from the most general and basic skills to the more specific. We will show later that training sessions are built around a basic goal theme, proceeding from easy to more difficult situations on that theme and in that session.

It is often the case that patients cannot or will not provide suitable social goals, or do not accept those that the therapist suggests, and some other therapeutic approach – particularly eclectic, brief insight psychotherapy – may be necessary before social skills training can commence. However, before patients are referred elsewhere, there are a number of practical techniques the therapist can use to try to help the patient overcome psychological blocks of this kind. In the case of conflict between desire for and fear of social encounters, a straightforward desensitisation approach may help, based on a hierarchy of social situations graded according to difficulty. In the case of depression, social needs may be suppressed to the point where they are no longer consciously acknowledged. In these cases we ask the patient to think of someone he admires and would like to resemble, and to specify those things the 'model' does that he (the patient) would like to do. Alternatively, we ask the patient to tick off a list of attributes, first for 'Me as I am' and secondly for 'Me as I'd like to be'. These probes often provide leads for exploration of goals.

CONTRACTS

Kanfer and Karoly (1972) have pointed out the importance and have demonstrated the effectiveness of obtaining a contract with, or 'intention statement' from, the patient or subject.

A promise made under contract enhances self-regulation of behaviour towards mutually agreed objectives and makes therapist rewards dependent on those objectives. The contract also alters the relationship from the doctor-patient kind to one of a client-specialist kind, where the continuation of therapy is conditional on both keeping their sides of the bargain.

The contract is used mainly for homework assignments. These assignments should be mutually agreed and written down on a suitable form (see Homework Report, p. 185) with the following specifications: (i) the guidepoints for succeeding in the task(s); (ii) the situation(s) in which the task(s) should take place (i.e. time, place, etc.); (iii) number of successes and failures; (iv) a description of what actually happened. The tasks given should be closely related to training and within the patient's capability. Finally, the therapist should reward only achievements and attempts, not promises.

GROUP AND INDIVIDUAL TREATMENT

Opinions differ about the 'mix' of patients, most favouring groups rather than individuals, larger (8 to 12) rather than smaller groups, and homogeneous rather than mixed groups.

The advantages of training in groups are:

(i) The group is a ready-made social situation in which participants undergoing training can practise on each other. It has the advantage of being 'real' rather than simulated, as individual sessions tend to be, and the chances of new social behaviour generalising to other social situations increase.

(ii) Group training makes considerably more economical use of therapists' time.

(iii) Patients tend to feel less intimidated in a group of people in a similar position to themselves. This is an important consideration in social skills training, which is necessarily directive and personal in nature.

Disadvantages of training in groups are:

(i) Members often show disturbed behaviour and provide bad models for each other. They may also develop skills for dealing with abnormal rather than normal behaviour.

(ii) There is a loss of flexibility often needed for concentration on an individual's particular problems.

There are also advantages and disadvantages of homogeneity in groups. In homogeneous groups the same training programme can be applied to everyone, but the patients may be uniformly passive and difficult to mobilise, and they do not function as good models for each other.

We suggest the following: Very disturbed or regressed patients should be given individual training with one therapist, using outside people, such as nurses, students or other volunteers as role-partners. Such patients may need a large number of sessions, and should eventually be placed in a group. Other patients can be put into groups of six with two therapists, which seems to us the best compromise in view of the above points, and the manual is presented with this number in mind.

The following two kinds of patients can be usefully mixed: Those with observable social skills deficits (socially inadequate) and those with competence in skills but whose performance is disrupted by anxiety (socially phobic). Social skills training is effective for both kinds of patients (Trower *et al.*, see reference p. 129) and works, we believe, in different but complementary ways, so that phobics can be active and useful models for the less adequate, while learning to cope with their own anxiety.

For some purposes, such as revision, reports, demonstration, etc., the members stay in one group, but for other tasks (imitation, practice, feedback) they divide into two 'work triads' (described on p. 182), each with a therapist.

Sessions should last no more than $1\frac{1}{2}$ hours at one session a week, or one hour at two sessions a week.

Training routine

The form of training sessions will vary according to the type of problems, but the following is a well-tried training 'package' for general use, upon which the sections of the manual are based and into which specialised techniques such as systematic desensitisation, guided participation, covert modelling etc. can be slotted where necessary. The general training package comprises the following (for a lengthier treatment of this, see Goldstein *et al.* 1976, or Liberman *et al.* 1975):

(a) The setting
(b) Revision of the previous session

(c) A single skill theme with a description of function, components and instruction in use

(d) A learning routine of demonstration, imitation, feedback, practice and guidance

(e) Homework assignments on the training sessions.

SETTING (figure 7.1)

Training can be usefully carried out with a minimum of facilities and equipment – single room, a few chairs, table and tape recorder. However, we have found the following set-up preferable: An observation room and a studio room are separated by a one-way screen. The studio room has all-round sound absorbing curtains and carpeting, good overhead lighting with one or two floodlights, hanging microphones, a large T.V. monitor with sound, three or more armchairs and some upright chairs, one large and one small table, a blackboard and a few props. The observation room contains most of the technical equipment, including a video system with two cameras – one for a wide, standard shot, the other with a zoom lens and monitor for close-ups and following the action. It also contains a tape recorder, speakers and T.V. monitor, and a press-button panel of counters and timers. Equipment also includes an ear microphone, which is simply a miniature headphone attached by a lead to an amplified microphone.

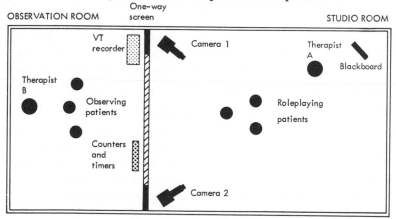

At the first training session, the patient or patients are shown over the studio set-up and given a demonstration. In group sessions, patients will be encouraged to operate the cameras and counters and timers.

REVISION

Each session, except the first, begins with a revision of the main points of the previous training session and a report from the patient on his successes and failures during the week. The therapist praises the patient for successes, and asks for information on the precise nature of failures (e.g. didn't do it because frightened, misperceived the cues, faulty response). This not only serves to minimise the importance of the failure, by narrowing it down to a particular fault, but provides the information for corrective training in the current session.

DESCRIPTION AND FUNCTION OF SKILLS TO BE TAUGHT

The therapist should take a single theme, such as some aspect of listening skill, because simplicity helps the patient acquire new knowledge. This theme is then analysed into a sequence of behavioural elements which serve as learning points and are written down and memorised. The therapist then helps the patient understand – by questioning and instruction – how this skills sequence functions in ordinary everyday interaction, the effect it produces in others and on the social life of the individual, and in particular how it will help the patient.

DEMONSTRATION, IMITATION, FEEDBACK,
PRACTICE AND GUIDANCE

This routine (i) shows the skill by demonstration, (ii) gets the patient to try it out by imitation, (iii) gives him feedback, including reinforcement, on the effect of his efforts, (iv) shapes his responses by practice, feedback and guidance.

Demonstration. To maximise the effect of demonstration the model should be *similar* to the patient in certain respects, particularly *age* and *sex*, and should be liked by the patient. The model should not give a *masterful* but rather a *coping* performance, showing he has difficulties but is nonetheless effective. The modelling should be clear cut, follow the learning points closely, and, if successful, the model himself should be rewarded by the therapist. It is best if more than one person models the skill in question, or if one model demonstrates two or more times. The patient is asked to follow the learning points as the demonstration proceeds. The demonstration may be shown live or on videotape. The former is more personal, dramatic and realistic, while the latter has the advantage of allowing careful preparation, can be replayed in whole or part, and saves on time and personnel. Ideally, video displays would be combined with live modelling by role partners or, in groups, by the better patients.

Imitation. The patient is invited to perform the same skill – to '*role-play*' the model. His first attempt should be as exact an imitation as possible (again to help him memorise the learning points) using the same or similar dialogue. If the patient finds the demonstration unconvincing, he can offer alternative suggestions, or alternative scenes can be tried. Suggestions for dealing with other problems are given later. In groups, some patients may be good at role-playing and serve as models.

Feedback. The therapist should praise the good aspects of the performance, focussing on the task and guidepoints rather than the person, to depersonalise the impact of his comments. This can be followed by audio or video feedback and an invitation to the patient to comment on his own performance, and to his role-partner to say what psychological impact the patient's performance had on him. In a group, other patients may give feedback at this stage. Evidence from some experiments (reviewed by Rosenthal 1974) shows that one of the most important factors in feedback is the amount of positive, as opposed to negative, comment. It is suggested that there should be proportionately more praise and positive expectations than criticisms.

Feedback should emphasise the effect rather than the appearance ('You made me feel you were not interested by looking away', rather than 'You looked bored . . .'). It should be *detailed* and *specific*, referring to actual movements, expressions, postures, etc., and also highly *focussed*, dealing with only those aspects relevant to the learning points and leaving other aspects until later. Other characteristics of effective feedback are: It should be concise, given as promptly as possible after the observed behaviour, in non-technical language, and should concentrate on behaviour over which the individual has some control.

Practice. From the feedback comments, a few correction points can be written down, and the patient practises these aspects of the scene in some detail and with continuous encouragement and guidance from the therapist. He is also invited to improvise more and more, making the responses 'his', as he progressively shapes the action into his own preferred style.

Imitation and practice serve two purposes. They enable the patient to acquire the skills taught, and they facilitate the application of these skills in real settings. The first of these is achieved as described above, by straightforward exercises in which they practise the steps laid down in the manual. The second is achieved by role-play 'simulations' of actual or possible real-life encounters in which they describe and allocate roles to other patients, or the therapists describe the situation, arrange props accordingly, and then act out their own role, introducing the new skills as appropriate. This helps to generalise the skills to real situations. This generalisation is reinforced by specifying homework assignments which are as similar as possible to the role-play simulations.

This routine can be effectively used in a 'work triad' of three patients guided by a therapist. Two of the patients can be given complementary participant roles, such as listener and speaker, while the third is a monitor. The participants learn the skill by working through the sequence of learning points, while the monitor learns by observation and teaches by giving feedback. Patients are moved around after three or four minutes so that each has experience in each role. A practical example of this is given in 'A Brief Conversation', pp. 186–9.

HOMEWORK ASSIGNMENTS

The homework assignments are an integral part of the training in that the patient can put into practice the skills learned during the therapy session. The ideal arrangement is as follows: The patient writes down on his Homework Report form the skills theme and the learning points. He suggests times, places and situations where he can put into practice the skill, and states his intention to do so. These situations may be graded according to difficulty, e.g. starting a conversation with a member of the family, a good friend, an acquaintance and, finally, a stranger. In groups, these commitments are made out loud and patients made answerable to each other to keep to them. (Suggested homework assignments have been included in that part of the Trainees' Handbook concerned with basic conversation, pp. 262–88).

In addition to the Homework Report, patients should also

List of social goals

Name: . . . .
Date: . . . .

A = Importance (0 = low, 10 = high)
B = Anxiety (0 = low, 10 = high)
C = Incompetence (0 = low, 10 = high)

Treatment Sessions

Goals	Before			1			3			5			7			9			After		
	A	B	C	A	B	C	A	B	C	A	B	C	A	B	C	A	B	C	A	B	C
1.																					
2.																					
3.																					
4.																					
5.																					
6.																					
7.																					
8.																					
9.																					
10.																					

keep a daily diary, in which they give a brief description of all social events they observed or participated in, and what they felt about them. The diaries are an important source of material for the training exercises.

Difficult cases

The training routine described above is particularly adaptable for helping both highly sensitive and insensitive patients, and increasing motivation generally.

Anxious and sensitive individuals can be helped in a number of ways, such as first reading from a script (preferably written by themselves) and trying to recall the script in subsequent rehearsals. Alternatively, such patients can begin in a fairly passive, non-participatory role and take a more active part as confidence grows. For instance, a patient may find it easier to begin as a monitor, giving feedback, then a prompter giving instructions and suggestions to another patient, perhaps through an ear-microphone while the action is going on, and finally become a full participant role-player. Another method is to send patients away to other rooms in groups of two or three with a clearly laid out task. This gives them the opportunity to prepare before exposing themselves to others. It may also be better to expose sensitive patients to a smaller group at first.

A patient who genuinely lacks sensitivity to feedback can learn from role-reversal, in which the therapist or patient adopting his role accentuates, if necessary, the deficits he displays. Video and audio feedback should be used early in the training with this kind of patient.

Motivation can often be increased by carrying out training in a game or 'workshop' form, for instance, guessing games in which patients decode each other's signals from only one channel – e.g. vocal expression of surprise, facial expression of disbelief. Signals or roles to be played or demonstrated can be taken from a hat or randomly chosen from a list. At a later stage of training patients can be encouraged to make their own scenarios on videotape, e.g. being interviewed, flirting, being assertive etc., taking turns at director, actor and cameraman. Two groups may be formed which work as competitive or cooperative teams, with one group making a film and keeping records from the observation room while the other group acts out a scene in the studio. Such exercises help create a 'workshop' as opposed to a clinical atmosphere – a difference in emphasis which is fundamental to social skills training philosophy.

Homework report

Name:
Date:

1. Homework assignment(s)

2. Guidepoints

3. Number of successes

4. Number of attempts

5. Description of what happened

6. Guidepoints used

References

BANDURA, A. (1969) *Principles of Behavior Modification.* New York: Holt, Rinehart & Winston.

GOLDSTEIN, A. P. (1973) *Structured Learning Therapy: Toward a Psychotherapy for the Poor.* New York and London: Academic Press.

GOLDSTEIN, A. P., SPRAFKIN, R. P. AND GERSHAW, N. J. (1976) *Skill Training for Community Living.* Oxford and New York: Pergamon Press.

KANFER, F. H. AND KAROLY, P. (1972) Self-control: A behavioristic excursion into the lion's den. *Behavior Therapy*, 3, 398–418.

KAZDIN, A. E. (1974) The effect of model identity and fear-relevant similarity on covert modeling. *Behavior Therapy*, 5, 624–35.

LIBERMAN, R. P., KING, L. W., DERISI, W. AND MCCANN, M. (1975) *Personal Effectiveness: Guiding People to Assert Themselves and Improve their Social Skills*. Chicago, Ill.: Research Press.

ROSENTHAL, R. (1974) On the social psychology of the self-fulfilling prophecy: Further evidence for Pygmalion effects and their mediating mechanisms. *Module 53*, 1–28. New York: MSS Modular Publications, Inc.

SHAPIRO, D. A. (1969) Empathy, warmth and genuineness in psychotherapy. *British Journal of Social & Clinical Psychology*, 8, 350–61.

2. Introductory skills

Briefing

The beginning of training is in many ways the most difficult and critical. Patients are often at their most vulnerable, negative and intolerant. The situation may bring out the worst features of their own problems. The therapists must be sure not to respond negatively, they must endeavour to prevent the training from becoming another failed experience, avoid raising patients' anxieties and yet present the training as practical and relevant. This section is therefore devoted to a highly structured yet simple and basic everyday skill that is directly related to social inadequacy. It can be used to facilitate group support and cohesion, and provides a conceptual framework for the training programme as a whole. In this section we give a step-by-step description of a brief conversation, adding to it and modifying it as the training progresses, and presenting it in the form of practical exercises.

Presentation

Patients are asked to sit round in a fairly small circle.

Therapist A: 'Many of the difficulties people have described are concerned with starting and maintaining conversations. Some can't start conversations, some can't think of things to say or they can't say things they want to say, some feel that nobody wants to talk to them. So we will begin with this: Starting, holding and ending a brief conversation. This is what we shall do: First, I shall explain the steps involved, second, we shall demonstrate those steps, third, we'll ask you to try it out and practise it here, fourth, we shall ask you to try it out with your own acquaintances. We think you will find it both easy and rewarding. We shall begin with very basic and very easy and simple steps, and then add things as we go along. To start with, then, turn to Exercise 1 [see Trainees' Handbook, p. 263] in your guidepoint booklet. The steps are:

First, turn to someone in your group

Second, greet him by name

Third, ask two questions

Fourth, answer any questions

Fifth, close conversation.

Now my colleague will describe a situation in which he bumps into an acquaintance at work but doesn't go through these five steps. You will see what happens when he *doesn't* go through them.'

Therapist B then describes a situation in which he passes a workmate in the corridor who starts to greet him but he does not respond. The workmate is rather taken aback and annoyed. The scene is role-played between the two therapists, or, preferably, between a patient and therapist, and should clearly demonstrate the effect of failure to use the routine (e.g. annoyance, irritation, surprise, etc.). The same scene in which the therapist goes through the five steps with his patient, is then re-enacted as in the following example:

First: looks, recognises, gives eyebrow flash of recognition

Second: greets, 'Hello, George.'

Third: asks two questions, 'How are you?' and 'How's the work going?'

Fourth: answers any questions, 'I'm fine.' 'Got a rush job on at the moment.'

Fifth: takes leave, 'Must get on. See you later. Cheers.'

Patients are asked for their comments on the different effects of the two role-plays, and to give comparable experiences of their own.

Therapist A then attempts to get all the patients to go through the 'brief conversation' as follows: he engages the nearest patient and works through the five steps (prompting the patient to provide him with questions for step four). This patient is then asked to turn to the next patient and work through the same routine. The second patient turns to the third and so on. The routine is then repeated, but in a more realistic role-play, with pairs of patients walking past each other in an imaginary corridor. Patients are then reseated, but in different positions. Video feedback is probably not advisable at this stage.

Therapist A congratulates the group on carrying out the task, and continues: 'We can add to or change this basic conversation to make it more relevant to the problems each of you have. First, do any of you feel that others are unfriendly and don't want to talk to you?' If the answer is yes, an example is asked for. 'That's one thing we can do: After recognition, look and see if the other is friendly and is ready to start a conversation. Second, does anyone feel that, during the conversation, the other person loses interest?' Again, examples are asked for. 'That's another thing we can do – show more interest, listen more carefully. Thirdly, does anyone feel he runs out of things to say?' 'That's something else we can do – disclose more information about ourselves. Let's change the brief conversation to include these extra things (Exercise 2):

Therapist B then demonstrates these steps in role-play as follows:

First: looks, gives eyebrow flash
Second: identifies other's attitude as positive – wants to talk; decides to go on
Third: 'Hello, George.'
Fourth: 'How are you?' 'How's the work going?' 'What are you doing exactly?'
Fifth,   he responds to the answers with:
          'Mhmm,' 'Yes,' 'Are You?' Nods head
Sixth: 'I'm fine.' 'Got a rush job on.'
Seventh: 'At the moment, I'm . . .' (give details of job)
Eighth: 'Must get on; see you later. Cheers.'

The patients are then divided up into triads, one as the initiator of the conversation, one as responder and one as monitor, the task of the monitor being to make sure that the initiator goes through all the steps. If this routine is carried out successfully, patients are encouraged to improvise their own brief conversations, filling in the blanks in Homework Assignment 1 using the basic steps as guidance.

Therapist B summarises: 'In the weeks that follow we will go into more detail to examine the skills involved in each of these steps. We will deal with those things we do in our heads and which we call observation skills – that is, looking at others, identifying their intentions and attitudes, taking in what they say. We will deal with those things we actually do, like listening skills, speaking skills and self-expression. Later still, we will deal with being warm and friendly, and with being assertive and influencing other people.' The homework assignment is then discussed and clarified and the session ended.

3. Observation skills

Briefing

Observation skills training should come early in the programme, since subsequent skills depend on it. It focusses on the information essential for social behaviour, it is a covert rather than overt activity and therefore less anxiety-arousing, and it focusses the patients' attention outside himself, thereby reversing a common habit and reducing self-consciousness. Observation training and related topics, such as perception and feedback, continue to feature in later sections which appropriate, e.g. listener skills. Putting observation training first should encourage a habit for all future social activity.

This section has two aims: first to sensitise patients to a wider range of social information, from facts about their neighbourhood to the small social cues such as the raising of eyebrows; second to use this information to arrive at impressions, judgments and other forms of decisions, and to check out the accuracy of these. We start with patients' own experiences and get them to do a number of exercises to get the maximum information out of these. For instance, we find some patients miss cues or block them out, and need to be taught what these cues are and how to observe more systematically. Or patients may perceive cues but interpret them inaccurately, and need to be shown how inferences and evaluations from behaviour are made – and often wrongly made. It should be emphasised that observation training is more effective in groups, as will become apparent.

Presentation

Therapist A: 'The aim of social skills training is to help people get into and be more effective in social situations. Like any other kind of skill, we need to start by having a good look at the problem, to look before we leap. We need to get into situations, to be good observers, to be able to size up situations and be good judges of others. What happens if we don't do these things? First, through remaining in isolated settings, we shall never have the opportunity to make social contacts and learn about people. Second, through lack of accurate information we won't know what to do in situations and may do the wrong thing or end up doing nothing at all. Third, we may judge people's feelings and attitudes wrongly and end up in unpleasant misunderstandings, or feel inadequate, nervous or rejected. To deal with the first point, everyone will have homework assignments to go to different places to meet and observe others. The aim of this session is to learn how to make accurate observations and realistic evaluations of what we see once we're in a situation. So, as a first step, I'd like to ask each of you to describe in general terms the nature of your difficulty, and to give one example. This is what we shall do. My colleague will give you an example, using the guidepoints in Exercise 3.'

Therapist B then describes a general problem such as talking to people he does not know very well. He then gives an example: He went to a party at which he vaguely knew two or three people, but could not get into conversation and stood in silence most of the time, before going home feeling miserable.

The patients are then asked to describe a problem and an example, drawing on their diaries if necessary (Exercise 3).

GETTING INFORMATION ABOUT THE SITUATION (Exercise 4)

Therapist A then continues as follows: 'For good social skills you need information, for two reasons. Firstly, you need information in order to have relevant things to talk about, and this includes facts about the situation and about the other people involved. Second, you need information about people's feelings and attitudes, and this includes their attitude to you. First let's have a look at the factual information you need. Look at the guidepoints in Exercise 4, as my colleague describes his situation in more detail.'

After the demonstration, patients are asked to follow suit, using the guidepoints.

GETTING INFORMATION ABOUT OTHER'S FEELINGS AND ATTITUDES (Exercise 5)

Therapist A continues: 'In addition to this factual information, we need to know what other people feel and believe, and we do this by observing what they do, and by checking our impressions with those of others. We now need a more detailed picture of the situation, and my colleague is going to try to recreate the situation he has already described.'

Therapist B (Peter) then enacts the party situation described earlier (other trainers usually prefer to think up their own situations):

Peter arrives at a private house party to which he has been invited by a work colleague. The guests are mostly standing. He looks around but sees no one he recognises, so he gets a drink from a nearby drinks table, and stands awkwardly by the table, feeling tense and looking sullen. Suddenly the host, John, appears, goes up to Peter and greets him cheerily and welcomes him to the party. Peter responds in a half-hearted way, says little, looks at the floor and out of the window, appearing to want to end the conversation. John looks a little uncomfortable and perplexed, but persists, suggesting he introduces Peter to the other guests, but Peter declines with a blunt 'no thanks'. The host now begins to look irritated, shrugs his shoulders and says, 'Oh well, it's up to you', and leaves.

The role-play simulation of such a situation should be carefully thought out and rehearsed by the therapists beforehand, to ensure it illustrates the steps in exercises 5 to 7. It can be video recorded, or acted live, or both.

In the case of live simulation, the second therapist arranges the furniture and any other props and selects and gives roles to patients and to the other therapist, to simulate the party situation. Various improvisations can be used in case of difficulty or refusal on the part of patients, such as the second therapist doubling roles.

However, the principal roles should be enacted by the therapists. The situation should ideally be one that the therapist recalls as participant or witness, since we found it extremely difficult to portray invented ones realistically. It should also be similar in kind to those experienced by the patients, such as difficulty in starting or maintaining a conversation (as in our example), or dealing with an assertive person. The role play should not last more than about two minutes and should be videotaped or at least tape-recorded if this wasn't done beforehand. The advantage of videotape is that the scene can be replayed and the action frozen, which facilitates observation of behavioural elements. The advantage of live simulation is that it may succeed in getting patients involved and accustomed to their image on television at a time when the focus of attention is not on themselves.

After the role play or viewing, the patients are referred to the guidepoints in Exercise 5 in the handbook, and therapist B describes his judgments and observation of the principal interactors in the role play, using the guidepoints as follows:

First,   Identifies individual(s) to be described

Second,   what attitude was the other expressing
        (a) in general
        (b) to therapist B?

Third,   how did therapist B get these impressions
        (goes through the social signals)?

Fourth,   did others agree with therapist B's impressions?
        The therapists ask each patient in turn to give his impressions of the individual being described. Invariably these impressions differ showing that alternatives can be equally or more valid. Therapist A then summarises these alternatives.

Fifth,   what alternative impressions might have been formed?

Sixth,   how sure is therapist B now about his first impression?

In detail, the exchange might go something like this:

Therapist A says to B: 'First point, you've identified someone – John, the host. The second point is, can you identify the attitudes John seems to be expressing?' Therapist B then gives an account which is inaccurate. For instance, while John appeared perplexed and irritated, therapist B interpreted him as rejecting and hostile.

Therapist A: 'The third point is: from what information did

you form this impression?' Therapist B goes through some of the elements, using the videotape replay for demonstration, e.g. 'He is orientated away, looks away, his face is angry, speaks briefly, long silences . . .'

Therapist A: 'The fourth point is, what do other people think John's attitude is?' He asks each of the patients in turn to give their impressions of John, and what information they based this on. Their impressions will differ to some extent, showing (fifth point) that alternatives can be equally or more valid.

Therapist A then says to B: 'The fifth point is, how sure are you now about John's attitude to you?' Therapist B then comments: 'I still think he was rather unfriendly, but not as much as I thought at first.' Patients are again invited to comment.

Therapist A then summarises as follows: 'We all form impressions and judgments about each other, but often get it wrong because of poor observation, misinterpretation and not getting other points of view. So my colleague made his judgment but without checking it out by careful observation of the social signals, and without checking it out with others. This exercise, then, is a checking out routine for making accurate observations. I would like each of you to try it now.' Each patient is asked to create a role-play simulation, and all these should be videotaped.

Role-play simulations are time-consuming, but time well spent, since the film will be used in subsequent sections, e.g. self-perception. In the case of refusals one must rely on reported observations.

CAUSES OF OTHER'S BEHAVIOUR (Exercise 6)

If the patient perceives the *message* correctly, he may yet misinterpret the *reason* for the other's behaviour, attributing it to the other's attitude towards himself. We describe three possible causes. Firstly, some behaviour is usually due more to the situation and the roles of the participants than to them as persons, e.g. happiness at a celebration, sadness at a funeral, or the friendliness of a salesman. Secondly, there is some behaviour which is due to the person's enduring personality style, rather than the behaviour of others. Or it may be due to the mood he is in. Third, it may be due to the behaviour of the particular person he is interacting with.

Therapist A says: 'We have looked at how problems can arise by mistaking the messages other people send us, and by responding on the basis of these wrong interpretations. So it is important to make accurate observations by using the check-out routine. But it is also important to know why he is expressing that feeling. First, the boss may treat you in a superior way, but then bosses usually treat employees in that way – it is their job, their role. We recognise this when we say, 'Oh, he was just doing his job; he had to do that'. If we don't ask why, we may take it personally, and that would be a mistake. A person is expected to be sad at a funeral, solemn at a cermony. If we don't ask why, we may think it is we who are making them feel sad or solemn, and that would also be a mistake. There are many other examples: policemen, doctors, bank managers, receptionists are expected to behave in an official and businesslike way – that does not mean they are being unfriendly. Even the man-in-the-street behaves rather formally to a stranger; indeed a friendly stranger arouses suspicion.

Secondly, a person may express anger or seem superior, but it may be due to his personality – he behaves that way to most people. If we don't ask why we may, again, take it personally, and that, too, would be a mistake. The same applies to a person in a bad mood – it may be caused by indigestion, a hangover, or losing money on the horses.

Thirdly, the feelings expressed by another may indeed be due to you, or another person. The next step in our check-out routine, then, is to ask why is he feeling that way – because of the situation, his personality, his mood, someone else or me?

My colleague will now tell us why people at his party behaved the way they did.' Therapist B then works through the guide-points in Exercise 6, and invites other patients to do the same for their situations, and suggests alternative reasons for the behavior of others.

SELF-OBSERVATION (Exercise 7)

Therapist A: 'We have looked at how you may form wrong impressions about others. Now let's look at how others may form wrong impressions about you. Let's have a look at the role-play situations which we previously filmed, this time focussing on your performance, and work through the steps in Exercise 7.'

Material for demonstrating this can come from the same videotapes made earlier. The videotape of therapist B's party scene can be used, attention now being focussed on therapist B's own performance. The five points in Exercise 8 are worked through, with therapist B again giving an account – this time of himself – which is obviously inaccurate, e.g. while he appears cold and withdrawn he thinks he is being friendly. Other patients give impressions which will, with guidance, underline this misperception. Therapist B gives an account of the elements of his behaviour, with contributions from the others, and finally comes to doubt that he looks friendly, saying: 'I wanted to be friendly, but it looks as if this did not come across very well.'

Patients are asked to contribute more situations, which are recorded, or earlier scenes are replayed on the videotape.

Video feedback in this exercise should be used with discretion. It is most effective with less sensitive patients, but should be omitted for extremely anxious and self-conscious individuals (Sarason and Ganzer 1973). In the latter case it is preferable to rely on reported observations and carefully handled feedback from others.

In this exercise the therapists are looking for patients' own observed discrepancy between intended and actual performance, and the behavioural elements underlying this. It is preferable to elicit their own observations, and to emphasise their effects on others rather than deficiency in themselves. The elements listed will be useful in later aspects of training. There is no need at this stage to make the list comprehensive – a few salient features are sufficient.

Therapist A continues: 'These examples have shown that if we don't want to be misunderstood, we have got to use the right social signals, and much of the training is designed to help do this.

'In summary, then, we have tried to show how we come to misunderstand each other: that we sometimes misinterpret the messages people send us, and that sometimes we send messages that are misinterpreted by others. Why is this bad? It is bad because if I wrongly think you are being unfriendly, then I might be unfriendly back, and this sets up a vicious circle – we each become more and more unfriendly, all because of misunderstandings. The same thing happens if you think I am being unfriendly.'

This is a convenient point to end the session, and to give Homework Assignment 2.

RECOGNITION OF EMOTIONS

So far the training has been on general principles of perception: how to be more aware of social cues, where to look for them and how to use them to check the accuracy of our inferences. We now move to the content of social behaviour and deal with the specific meaning of behavioural elements. We shall focus on the expression of emotion in the face and voice and the expression of attitudes in these and other areas of the body. Some of this information has already been discussed earlier in this book, and reference should be made to that. We shall deal here with the practical application of this material.

Face

There are six emotions which are found to be primary, in that other emotions are blends of these. The therapists should familiarise themselves with the facial elements of these and learn to encode them, and blends of them, from the training manual by Ekman and Friesen (1975). Photographs of the six emotions and the neutral face should be distributed to patients.

Therapist A: 'We have looked at the social signals we use, and what this means. But we can get much more information from these social signals. First, we shall learn how to read people's faces better – and this will also help us to be more expressive. These photographs (p. 269) show the six main emotions and a neutral face. Let's look closely at these faces, and later look at how more subtle expressions are formed.' Patients are referred to the list of face cues in Exercise 8 and a description of each expression is given as follows: Therapist A takes one of the photographs and points out the features of the three facial regions, namely brows/forehead, eyes/lids and lower face. He then asks the patients to identify features in the other photographs, by asking each patient to identify the emotion and the elements comprising it. Therapist A then points out that some emotions are expressed using only one or two elements, and do not involve the whole face. By way of illustration, Therapist B encodes just one or two elements from each emotion, leaving the rest of the face blank, e.g. surprise brow only, happy mouth only, fear brow and mouth only. Patients are again asked to identify the elements, and to comment on the effect of the partial expression. Finally, therapist A points out that some expressions are blends of two emotions. The second therapist again demonstrates, e.g. anger/happiness with anger brow and happy mouth; fear/surprise with fear brow and eyes, and surprise mouth. Patients identify the blends and elements, and comment on the effect.

Patients can now be divided into pairs or threes, one of whom will be an encoder, the others decoders. The encoders choose a full emotion expression, then a partial emotion expression, and finally a blend, while the decoders guess at the expressions formed. It is best at first to write out these tasks for the encoders on slips of paper. Also, for doing blends write down each facial element on a card and get the encoder to pick up two of these from a hat and express them.

This exercise may have to be postponed with some difficult groups and delayed until after listener and speaker skills, at which point they should have more confidence. After the exercise, therapist A says: 'During the week try to recognise the expressions people use and note down the facial elements. Notice how people try to camouflage their emotions and note how their feelings leak out. Here are some tips:

What is the social situation? Is the person acknowledging mixed feelings? Is he denying being afraid? What does his body show? What is he expected to do in this situation? What do others think?

Watch out for what people do in the region around the eyes. They usually control this area less well than the lower part of the face.

Notice the timing of the expression. How long does it take for the expression to appear (onset time), to remain before fading (duration), and to disappear (offset time).

Notice if the expression fits with what is being said.

Notice fleeting expressions which may give the game away before being controlled.

Finally, notice hand and foot movements, especially self-adaptators (scratching, etc.).

(For more information on this see 'Unmasking the Face', p. 200.)

Voice

The same format can be used for emotion expression in the voice, with the second therapist modelling in the same way, before patients try the encoding-decoding game (using the guide-points in Exercise 9), perhaps by reading extracts from printed material in the appropriate voice element.

After patients have a reasonable grasp of voice elements, face and voice cues can be used together, first in synchrony, where the face and voice elements are used to depict the same emotion, and secondly in the form of vocal-facial blends, where the face elements from one emotion and the voice elements from another are expressed together.

RECOGNITION OF ATTITUDES

Videotaped sketches of the two main interpersonal attitudes, friendly-unfriendly and assertive-submissive, should be prepared beforehand. In the following examples, we keep the situation the same, and vary the attitude of one of the participants, being sure to include the elements listed under Exercise 10. For instance, Mary is disclosing information and feelings about some recent problem at work. The sketches begin with John and Mary walking into the picture and then sitting down, John positioning his seat in accordance with the attitude to be expressed.

Videotaped sketches are clearly preferable to either static impressions or impromptu sketches, because attitudes, unlike emotions, are interactional, and videotape is a permanent record which can be replayed or 'frozen'. If no videotape equipment is available, impromptu sketches by the therapists should be pre-pared beforehand.

Sketch 1. John is expressing a warm attitude non-verbally, and is verbally supportive and positive.

Sketch 2. John is expressing a cold attitude non-verbally, and verbally gives little feedback or disclosure and meshes poorly.

Sketch 3. John is being dominant, giving advice, asking questions, interrupting and disclosing his own competence and superior life-style.

Sketch 4. John is being submissive, gives too much attention feedback (but not reflections) and agrees too often.

Sketch 5. John is being both friendly and assertive.

Therapist A: 'In addition to expressing (or concealing) their own feelings, people also express their attitudes to others verbally and non-verbally. Expressions of feelings show a person's subjective emotional state. But expressions of attitudes show what he thinks of the other person and the relationship between them. Let's now turn to the social signals which tell us what the other person's (and our own) attitude is.

'There are two important attitudes (or styles). First, there is friendliness (including warmth) – as against unfriendliness (including hostility, coldness and so on). Secondly, there is assertiveness (including strength and dominance) – as against submissiveness (including weakness, compliance etc.). To make you familiar with the cues which comprise each of these attitudes, we will play you a film in which these attitudes are expressed.

'In these sketches, John and Mary are having a conversation. In each one John expresses a different attitude to Mary. After each sketch we shall stop and ask you to identify from the list what attitude he was expressing.'

After this, Exercise 10 is practised (though this exercise, too, may have to be postponed). This is a convenient session endpoint, and Homework Assignment 3 can be given.

PROBLEM OF GAZE AVERSION

Many patients avert their gaze in social interaction, and if this persists, it will obviously undermine observation training. It is preferable to avoid direct training in looking, since this makes for self-consciousness and exacerbates feelings of inadequacy. We prefer to achieve the same objective by indirect means, such as the preceding exercises, e.g. close observation of the other's face. However, if gaze aversion persists, direct training may have to be attempted. We have found the following technique successful in some cases:

The patient is trained in relaxation. While relaxed, he is instructed to look at the other person for brief periods while the other looks away. This is followed by brief periods of mutual gaze alternating breaking gaze first or last. Looking time is slowly lengthened, until 2 or 3 second bursts can be achieved. He should then attempt much longer periods of looking while listening, and shorter bursts of looking while speaking.

In severe cases of gaze phobia, where eye-watering, blushing etc. occur, imaginal desensitisation should be tried before each practice session.

References

ARGYLE, M. (1969) *Social Interaction*. London: Methuen.
DAVITZ, J. R. (1964) *The Communication of Emotional Meaning*. New York: McGraw Hill.
EKMAN, P. AND FRIESEN, W. V. (1975) *Unmasking the Face : A Guide to Recognising Emotion from Facial Expressions*. New York: Prentice-Hall.
MEHRABIAN, A. (1972) *Nonverbal Communication*, Chicago, Ill.: Aldine Atherton.
SARASON, I. G. AND GANZER, V. J. (1973) Modeling and group discussion in the rehabilitation of juvenile delinquents. *Journal of Counseling Psychology*, 20, 442–9.

4. Listening skills

Briefing

Listener skills training continues the emphasis on orientation to the other person and is a good beginning for performance skills, both in terms of difficulty (being rather more passive than active) and in terms of logical sequence linking perception and performance skills.

The section is concerned largely with responses to mainly explicit conversation and is divided into four subsections: (a) *Verbal and non-verbal reflections*. These involve the accurate perception (decoding) of the emotional and factual content of the speaker's utterances and reflecting back to the speaker (encoding) of this content in a summarising statement. This bridges both perception and performance skills. The reflection communicates both comprehension and empathy, involves the psychological processes of 'taking the role of the other' and reinforces speaker disclosures (Truax and Carkhuff 1967; Vitalo 1971; Sarbin and Allen 1969). (b) *Attention feedback*. This involves small, minimal response cues which signal attention and comprehension and also reinforce the speaker's utterances (Williams 1964). (c) *Commentary*. These are responses which communicate the listener's own beliefs, opinions, etc. about the speaker's utterances and often produce a change in the speaker's subsequent utterances.

(d) *Questions*. These start, maintain and change the speaker's utterances and are used for getting information.

It will be seen from the above that listening involves both perception and performance components. We have found it useful in training to have three sets of videotape sketches of the expression of the six primary emotions (two examples of each emotion), being sure to include some of the behavioural elements which characterise them. Here are six suggested sketches, in each of which a primary emotion is expressed verbally and non-verbally about an anecdotal experience. (Shots should be full front with the actor apparently speaking to the viewer and need be no longer than 20 seconds.)

Sketch A. John is reporting how *surprised* he was to see how many new buildings, roads, etc. had sprung up in a town he recently visited.

Sketch B. Mary is a bus conductress and telling a story about how *fearful* she was when a group of drunken youths got on the bus and tried to cause trouble.

Sketch C. John is saying how *angry* he was because of bad servicing of his car.

Sketch D. Mary is telling about her *disgust* over a workmate's manners, e.g. when eating.

Sketch E. John is saying how *sad* he was when he heard his friend's marriage had broken up.

Sketch F. Mary is reporting how *happy* she is about a new outfit of clothes.

The second set of sketches should be subtler and more complex versions of these – either milder, or blends of two primary emotions. A list of these subtler emotions is given on page 204; for instance, in Sketch A, John may express curiosity rather than surprise, or a blend of surprise and anger.

We have also found it useful to prepare a list of ideal reflections to each of these sketches, e.g. (Sketch A) You were surprised because so much of the city had changed; (Sketch B) You felt frightened because the youths were causing trouble.

Presentation
'We have seen how we go wrong in interpreting what other people say to us, how this can lead to problems in a relationship, and

what steps we can take to become better observers. There are many reasons why we need this skill. First and foremost, we need it to be good listeners – and that is the topic of this session.

'When people talk they often tell us how they think, feel and believe and listeners usually respond to this – so that is the *first step* – identify the feelings, belief or opinion expressed.

'Now, as listeners we can respond in at least three ways to all this. One way is to *say back* the gist of what's said, e.g. "You say you feel . . . (feeling) because . . . (reason)." *Or* you can just nod your head etc., *or* you can comment and perhaps ask questions. We shall see how important these are in getting the speaker to talk more (or less). We shall deal with each of these in turn. Let's begin with the first one, saying back what was said, or what we call reflecting.'

REFLECTION

Verbal

This subsection is begun by therapist B demonstrating. He watches the first sketch and goes through the three reflection steps (Exercise 11):

First, The *feeling expressed* is surprise;

Second, The *reason* for his surprise is the number of new buildings which have sprung up;

Third, My reflection, therefore, is 'You feel surprised at the number of new buildings in the city.'

The next sketch is shown and a patient asked to respond in a similar way, using guidepoints in Exercise 11. After the first six emotion sketches have been worked through, therapist A says: 'That was very good. You recognised and reflected back the six primary emotions. We call these primary because all other emotions are derived from them. Now, I would be glad if each of you would tell an anecdote from your diaries in which you express a feeling about something, and then someone else would recognise and reflect it.' The anecdotes can include opinions and beliefs which usually contain emotional overtones.

Inevitably, some patients will have shown some inaccuracies in reflection, and this provides a lead into the next stage: Use of NV signals in increasing accuracy of emotion recognition.

Non-Verbal (Exercise 12)

Therapist A says: 'It is not always easy to be accurate about the second step – identifying the feelings expressed. How can we be more certain, more accurate? So far we have only looked at what people *say* their feeling is, but you will remember we can also *see* what their emotion is – by their non-verbal behaviour. What we can do now, therefore, is to look again at the non-verbal elements of emotion expression. Let's take the face and voice. We will play through the scenes on the videotape again and my colleague will *identify the feelings expressed*, the *non-verbal elements*, the *reason* for his feeling that way, and finally give a reflection.'

Patients are urged to ask themselves the questions listed in Exercise 12: 'CUES TO LISTEN AND LOOK FOR'.

Another videotape sketch is then played, and therapist B goes through the steps, amended as follows:

First, The feeling expressed is . . . .

Second, The elements of his expression are . . . (goes through list of face and voice cues)

Third, The reason for his feeling is . . .

Fourth, My reflection is . . . .

The rest of the sketches are shown and patients in turn are asked to go through the steps given in Exercise 12, using the lists of face and voice cues as guidance for step two. Various modifications can be made to simplify the task, such as playing back sound only and focussing on voice cues, or playing back vision only for face cues. Therapist A then says: 'You all did well – you picked up the non-verbal cues and made more accurate reflections. Now I would be glad if you would again tell an anecdote – the same or a different one – in which you express a feeling *non-verbally* and not verbally, and see if others can identify it *just* from non-verbal cues.'

Moodmatching (Exercise 13)

'Now there are two more things we can do to improve our reflections – one is to respond *non-verbally*, e.g. match a soft voice with a like response, and the other is to choose the right words.

'The first of these we will call *"mood matching"*. A listener is is seen as responsive and rewarding if he, for instance, matches a speaker's happy expression with a happy response. This is really the same as a reflection, only this time a non-verbal one. This is a very easy step – you just do what the speaker does. If the speaker smiles and speaks fast, you smile and speak fast too.' Therapist B then demonstrates, and patients practise either with tapes or with spontaneously produced sketches using the guide-points in Exercise 13. Guidance is given as to when *not* to use mood matching, in particular not matching depressed behaviour with depressive responses.

Verbal accuracy (Exercise 14)
Training in verbal accuracy can be presented as follows: 'You have done well in recognising emotions, but one problem we still have is finding the right words for these emotions. For instance, the other may not express fear so much as worry, anger so much as irritation. My colleague will now demonstrate a way of finding the right word. The technique is: identify the *general* feeling, then identify the *particular* feeling.'

Therapist B then watches a further video sketch (second series) and shows how to use the following categories to find the right word:

General:	*Anger*	*Happiness*	*Sadness*	*Fear*	*Disgust*	*Surprise/Interest*
	Annoyed	Pleased	Disappointed	Anxious	Contemptuous	Amazed
	Enraged	Satisfied	Sorry	Alarmed	Sickened	Curious
Particular:	Irritated	Relieved	Hurt	Worried	Shocked	Intrigued
		Delighted	Regretful	Uncertain		Fascinated
				Confused		

Thus, for example, after the first sketch, therapist B identifies the *general* feeling – say, surprise – and then the *particular* feeling – curiosity. Also, patients should try to identify the expressive non-verbal elements of these subtler emotions, e.g. the fear brow in an otherwise neutral face in worry, disgust face with closed mouth in contempt, anger brow in a neutral face in perplexity, etc. Patients are also urged to identify verbally and non-verbally blended feelings, for example:

Surprise/Disgust   Surprise/Fear   Happiness/Disgust
 =Shocked   =Apprehensive   =Scornful

Happiness/Sadness   Sadness/Anger
 =Melancholy   =Sulky

The practice routine in Exercise 16 is followed as before.

A final point on reflections. The therapists should insist on the use of the response frame: 'You feel ... because ... , until patients have mastered the principle, and they should *then be encouraged to generate their own spontaneous reflections*, using their own words.

ATTENTION FEEDBACK (Exercise 15)

Briefing
Listener responses may be placed on a continuum from full reflections at one end to attention feedback – or minimal responses (head nods, 'Mhmms', 'yes's') – at the other, with 'token' reflections ('I know what you mean', 'I see', 'I'm with you') in the middle. They are all, in a sense, reflections because they include the message that the listener is decoding the speaker's message, but vary in the extent to which this is explicit, as in reflections, or implicit, as in attention feedback. This section deals with attention feedback and 'token' reflections.

Presentation
'Up to now we have just dealt with reflections – saying back the gist of the speaker's message – and these are very important because they tell the speaker that you understand and care, and this is very rewarding to him. But of course we don't do this all the time in ordinary conversation. In fact, more often we will simply nod the head, say "mhmm", or "yeah" or "I see" or "I understand". In fact they all mean 'I understand' and are just abbreviated forms of reflections. They, too, are very important and rewarding to the speaker, and, in general, the more you use them, the more he will tell you, and vice versa. The first step, then, is to give a variety of responses as follows:' (write on blackboard)

Small responses	Head nod 'Mhmm' 'Yeah'
Medium responses	'I see' 'I know what you mean'
Full responses (reflections)	'You feel . . . because . . .'

'The second step is to make the responses at the right time, namely when the speaker wants it. The speaker lets us know when he wants this feedback by turning and looking at us when he makes a point or when he pauses. So the two steps are (1) give a variety of responses and (2) make them when the speaker looks up. We will demonstrate.'

Therapist A then talks for an extended period, disclosing one feeling. Therapist B uses all six responses, listed above and in Exercise 15, at the points when therapist A looks at him, being sure to use the reflection after the feeling disclosure. A variety of exercises (e.g. Exercise 15) can then be given to the patients, including getting each in turn to take the place of the therapist B, to talk in pairs or triads, or getting three patients to film the other three and vice versa.

Corrective feedback should also be given. It is particularly useful in this exercise to play back tapes and stop at the points where faulty responses are made. A better response is formulated – by therapists or patients – and this is rehearsed. Common deficiencies at this stage are: A patient misses an opportunity for a full reflection, or gives one inaccurately; a patient fails to use attention feedback, or uses it at the wrong time; a patient uses the wrong kind of response, e.g. rapid head-nods (which are usually interpreted as a bid to take up the conversation) instead of one or two slower ones.

This is a convenient session end-point, and Homework Assignment 4 should be given.

LISTENER COMMENTARY (Exercise 16)

Briefing
This section deals with the disclosure of the listener's own feelings, thoughts and beliefs *about* the speaker's message, as opposed to the focus of the previous sections on reflecting back the speaker's feelings etc. Theoretically, it is somewhat arbitrary whether this should be classified as a listener or speaker skill, but practically, it is a convenient point to introduce this change of emphasis and provides a lead into the more demanding sections on speaker skills.

Presentation
'So far, we have only learned to reflect back what people say. But

as listeners we have our own thoughts and feelings about what people say – sometimes we feel the same way, sometimes we don't. First, we must distinguish between *reflection* and *disclosure*. In the following exercise (Exercise 16), instead of reflecting "You feel . . . because . . ." we shall disclose "I feel (would feel) . . . because . . .". Second, we must distinguish between disclosures which are *similar to* or *different from* the speaker's. Third, we can choose between making our disclosures verbally, non-verbally or – preferably – both.'

The therapists then demonstrate these three points. Therapist A discloses feelings and opinions about his experiences. Therapist B then discloses how he would feel in those situations, alternating between feelings of similarity ('I would feel the same . . . ') and feelings of difference ('I would feel different'). In the latter case, for example, therapist A may express anger about juvenile delinquency, while therapist B may express sadness, surprise or disgust.

A variation is for therapist B to give a double response, combining a reflection and a disclosure, viz: 'You feel (believe, think) . . . , but I feel (believe, think) . . .'. Or therapist B discloses a different feeling from that expressed by the other by selecting a different facial expression or vocalisation. This can be demonstrated by listener 'mismatching', e.g. frowning to the speaker's smile, smiling to the speaker's expression of disgust, and so on. Other non-verbal listener responses include: raising of the brow (surprise) for a few seconds, with the rest of the face neutral, meaning doubt or questioning; if accompanied by a head movement sideways or backwards, it is an exclamation; if the surprise brow is accompanied by a disgust mouth, the meaning changes to sceptical disbelief; if a surprise brow and eyes are combined with a happy mouth, this may mean enthusiasm. Patients take it in turn to be listener and speaker in practising the production and recognition of these expressions, and expressors should be encouraged to think up as many alternative disclosures as possible.

Some of the non-verbal cues which may form part of the listener's commentary may be summarised as follows:

Agree	Nodding, smiling mouth
Disagree	Shaking head, lowered brow
Pleased	Surprise brow and eyes, happy mouth

Displeased	Lowered brow, anger or disgust mouth
Understand	Nodding, neutral face
Puzzled	Lowered brow, head to side
Surprised	Raised brow, wide eyes, lips parted
Interested	Slight raising of brows and eye widening, forward lean, erect tonus
Bored	Brow and upper eyelid lowered, mouth corner down, gaze lowered, low body tonus

QUESTIONS (Exercise 18)

Briefing

Question asking continues the change of emphasis from the more passive listener role to one requiring more initiative, and taking responsibility for maintaining and directing conversations. We introduce three different kinds of questions and a number of topics which these questions can be about. Much of the information gained from these questions can also be used in subsequent homework assignments.

Presentation

'So far, we have learned a range of listener skills which can be used to get other people talking more. But sometimes we have got to get people *started* and give them things to talk about, and to do this we usually ask questions. In this exercise we shall deal with various kinds of questions.

'First, we can ask very *general* or very *specific* questions. General questions such as "How are you?" "How are things going?" "What have you been doing recently?" allow the speaker to talk about something of his own choosing and are useful in getting the conversation started. Specific questions, such as 'Where did you go exactly?' 'What did you do exactly?', usually follow the general ones and are useful in getting and keeping the other going.

'Second, questions can be asked about *facts* and *feelings*. Fact-seeking questions such as "What did you do last weekend?" are used to get information and introduce new topics of conversation. Emotion and opinion-seeking questions include "What did you feel (think, etc.) about that?" "Did you . . . (enjoy, like) that?" "Were you . . . (annoyed, surprised) about that?" They are used to get others to self-disclose and usually follow fact-seeking questions.

'Third, questions can be *open* or *closed*. Open questions, like "What did you do at the weekend?" "Tell me more about that", cannot be answered with a yes or no, and they are useful for getting people to give fuller and more specific answers and therefore to talk more. Closed questions, like "Did you have a nice weekend?", on the other hand, can be answered with a yes or no and don't invite long answers.'

These three types of questions are then written on the black-board and patients referred to Exercise 18. The therapists then demonstrate them and patients are asked to practise them long enough to become familiar with their functional difference.

The use of Exercise 18 is outlined as follows:

First step: Ask your partner a general question (a) about the first topic (1).

Second step: Ask your partner a specific question (b) about the first topic (1). Ask more specific questions if you don't get enough information.

Third step: Ask your partner a feeling question (c) about the first topic (1).

The therapists demonstrate and the patients follow suit, being reminded to ask open questions whenever possible. In summary, therapist A says: 'This is a common question routine, and it is helpful to remember it as the GSF routine (general-specific-feeling). You can make up different orders and routines and we shall be doing this next time.'

Problems

Sometimes patients may be reluctant and anxious about asking questions. Reassurance ('People feel you are interested in them if you ask questions'), continual feedback from others ('Did you mind being asked questions?') and role reversal may help, or relaxation with a list of graded questions can be used in difficult cases. Also, patients may fail to use the appropriate NV accompaniments, and these should be practised, e.g. rising or lowering inflection on the last syllable, head movement, rapid brow raise. Further, some patients may over-use or misuse questions, and steps should be taken to avoid intimate questions, which may be rude or too challenging of others' behaviour or beliefs.

Revision

It is advisable at this point in training to have a session devoted to revision and integration of perception and listener skills. We take as a framework an elaborated version of the basic conversation referred to in the introduction.

Presentation

'Today we shall practise all the skills covered so far. We will put these together to make complete conversations, rather like we did in the introductory session. We shall practise the role of listeners in this exercise, and our task will be to get the other person to speak as much as possible.

'In a conversation there are two kinds of things we have to do. We have to make decisions and we have to carry out actions. We have to decide what messages other people are sending us and what we should do. Then we have to carry out some action on that decision. We have prepared a conversation routine consisting of several steps, each step consisting of a decision and an action. We will demonstrate this routine and then invite you to build conversations of your own and try them out.'

A conversation routine is given in Exercise 19. The therapists work through this routine and patients are asked to do the same, working with the aid of the guidepoints in Exercise 19.

This exercise can be organised as follows: One patient (A) is nominated to begin. He then secretly picks someone (B) from the rest of the group, and forms an opinion about him (Step 1). Patient A then goes to the observation room with one of the therapists, who is his confidante, and observes B interacting with the others, noting the elements of B's behaviour and his general style. He also notes the attitudes of the others towards B, and decides how much of B's behaviour is due to the situation, his personality and mood and to the others present in the room. He then checks and if necessary corrects his original judgment, with the help of the therapist (Step 2). Next, he decides on his own style, notes his feelings and prepares his behaviour (Step 3). He then goes into the main room, and during the ensuing interaction

(Steps 4 to 13) monitors his own performance (checks he is giving out the messages he intends and which are appropriate). He also monitors the other's performance, attending closely to his conversation and non-verbal style. After A has worked through all 13 steps, he is given the usual guided feedback, emphasising the effect of his behaviour. He is also asked to report on his own initial and continuing judgments. A second patient is then nominated, and the exercise repeated. Patients are then asked to construct their own spontaneous conversation routines with the above as guidance. This becomes an ongoing exercise during a conversation and for learning purposes it is often helpful to allow patients to pause at each decision point. The interaction can be speeded up in subsequent rehearsals. Finally, working in triads, the participants work without the aid of their guidepoints, the listener participant attempting to use as many techniques as possible to get the maximum verbal output from the speaker. An outside stooge may be brought in at some point and patients compete in getting the most speech from him within a given time. Useful feedback can be obtained from tape-recordings or from the monitors who check the number and variety of listener responses.

This is a convenient session end-point, and Homework Assignment 5 can be given.

References

CONDON, W. S. AND OGSTON W. D. (1966) Sound-film analysis of normal and pathological behavior patterns. *J. Nerv. and Ment. Dis.*, 143, 338–47.

EKMAN P. AND FRIESEN, W. V. (1975) *Unmasking the Face: A Guide to Recognizing Emotion from Facial Expressions.* New Jersey: Prentice-Hall, Inc.

SARBIN, T. R. AND ALLEN, V. L. (1969) Role Theory. In G. Lindzey and E. Aronson (eds) *Handbook of Social Psychology*, Vol. 1, Reading, Mass: Addison-Wesley.

TRUAX, C. B. AND CARKHUFF R. R. (1967), *Toward Effective Counseling and Psychotherapy*, Chicago, Ill.: Aldine.

VITALO, R. L. (1971) Teaching improved interpersonal functioning as a preferred mode of treatment. *Journal of Clinical Psychology*, 27, 166–71

WILLIAMS, J. H. (1964) Conditioning of verbalization: a review. *Psychological Bulletin*, 62, 383–93.

5. Speaking skills

Basic training

Briefing

Speaking skills are in some respects the mirror image of listening skills and patients should be familiar with the steps, having already experienced them indirectly as role-partners in the listening exercises. From now on, patients can increasingly take over the role of mutual trainers, helping each other to talk more, give the right responses, and so on. Research shows that unassertive trainees are very good at this. Flowers and Guerra (1974) showed that unassertive probation officers learned better from fellow-trainees than from professional instructors. Our experience is that this is often true for unassertive patients.

Presentation

'So far, we have concentrated on our role as listeners and some of the skills involved. To hold a conversation, we also need speaking skills, and this is what we shall now turn to.

'What, as speakers, should we put into our conversations? We shall mention two important things for ordinary social conversation: (a) There is factual information – about work, home, friends, day-to-day events and so on. (b) There are our opinions, beliefs and feelings about those things that we experience. Let's take factual information first.'

DISCLOSURE OF FACTUAL INFORMATION (Exercise 20)
'There are three points to remember. (i) We need a number of things to talk about. We have given in Exercise 20 a short list of topics with examples (already familiar to you as questioners – Exercise 18). (ii) We need to have done some of these things or have experience or knowledge of them. As part of your homework assignments you have already had experience of some of these topics. We will continue to give you assignments to help broaden your list of topics. (iii) We must be able to remember this information when we are talking. It will help you to remember things you have experienced if you write them down in your diaries soon after they have happened, and use this to prompt yourself in the

conversation you have here. Again, this is something you have already done and we will ask you to carry on doing it.'

These three points are written on the blackboard:

(i) Things to talk about
(ii) Experience and knowledge of them
(iii) Remembering the information.

Patients turn to the list: 'Conversation – Topics and Examples', in Exercise 20.

The question list in Exercise 18 follows the same sequence and the two lists can be used together in a question-answer conversation. The therapists demonstrate this, the first therapist working through the question list and the second through the conversation list. Patients work through the same question-answer routine, questioners being encouraged to probe and elicit as much information as they can. Speakers are encouraged to take their time and consult their diary forms for information and to be prepared to answer questions on any of the topics listed.

GENERAL V. SPECIFIC DISCLOSURES (Exercise 21)
Therapist A continues: 'In ordinary social conversation we usually move from general things to the details. For instance, "I went away for the weekend" is a general statement we might start with. Then we can go into more details – on the journey itself, where we went, whom we met, what we did. We start with a general statement to (a) put the listener in the picture, (b) see if he is interested anyway. If he is interested we give more details, because the listener needs more information and the details are intrinsically more interesting and will hold his attention.'

The following example is written on the blackboard and the therapists demonstrate it:

TOPIC	EXAMPLE
Anything you have been involved in recently.	*General :* 'Went away for the weekend/day.'
	Detail : Describe journey, place visited, things you did.

After the demonstration, the therapists choose the most conversationally retarded patients and probe for information, helping them, by successive rehearsals, to string together bits of information into a continuous utterance. The patients then try this (Exercise 21), reversing questioning and answering role, periodically.

The daily information patients collect in their diaries can be used in speaking skills training. Such descriptions can be read at first, and then told from memory. Questioners can again probe the speaker for comprehensive information.

It will become obvious from this session that some patients are lacking in point two – no experience of certain activities. These areas should be noted for inclusion as homework assignments at the end of the session.

FEELING DISCLOSURES

(i) Verbal (Exercise 22). Therapist A: 'As speakers in daily social conversations we tell people about things we have done and experienced – and we have practised that. In addition, we also tell people what we think, feel and believe about all those things. For instance, "I went away for the weekend" is information. "Had a lovely time" is a feeling. To practise disclosing our feelings, this is what we will do. First, take a topic from your list. Second, decide what you feel about it (the emotion categories in Exercise 15 can be used to help). Third, *describe it from that point of view*, being sure to use the appropriate word to describe your feeling.'

Patients are referred to Exercise 22. Therapist B then demonstrates. For example, 'I had a really *great* weekend. Went down to Bristol and met some friends I had not seen for years. It was *really nice* seeing them after all that time. We used to have some *good* times together', etc. Exercise 20 (speaking) and 18 (questioning) are fully complementary and patients can again combine them in a question-answer conversation.

(ii) Non-verbal (Exercise 23). This subsection is devoted to facial and vocal emotion expression and is for some patients the most difficult part of the training. If they have not already done so, patients should complete, or if necessary repeat, the encoding/decoding 'game' in Exercises 9 and 10 (observation skills), in which the encoder expresses a primary emotion, facially and vocally, and the decoder identifies the emotion expressed and lists the elements the speaker is using. This teaches the emotion cues, gives the speaker feedback on the success or failure of his expression and helps him learn the appropriate cues. This subsection teaches the use of these cues in the general conversation stream. Patients should use anecdotal experiences from the topics list.

The subsection is presented as follows: 'We can make it clear to the listener what we feel by telling him. We can make it clearer still – and more interesting – by showing him. We have already learned how to use the face and voice in expressing what we feel. Now let's practice using these in a conversation' (Exercise 23).

The role-partner or monitor then identifies the emotions expressed and their elements, viz.:

Emotion expressed: Surprise

Face cues: Brows raised, eyes wide, mouth open

Voice cues: High varied pitch, fast pace, rising tone.

After the usual demonstration, each patient in turn goes through all six emotions and blends of these in similar exercises, using the list from Exercise 15 as a prompt.

Therapists should bear in mind in this section that some emotions are best not expressed in some situations and cultures. The emphasis is on the expression of emotions in socially sanctioned ways, not on the release of emotional tension.

Additional training

NON-VERBAL DEFICITS

Direct training in particular non-verbal deficits has been left to this late stage because this is a particularly demoralising form of training, and if approached indirectly, as in the preceding sections, it may not in fact be necessary to confront the patient directly, with the risk of withdrawal and refusal. It is also essential to establish conversation first, since most N.V.C. depends upon and accompanies V.C.

Patients vary greatly in their particular non-verbal deficits, and for reasons of space we offer only a few guidelines, for training in two of the more important and complex elements – face and voice. More information on the description of non-verbal elements can be obtained from the rating scale guide or the texts listed at the end of this section.

Training for non-verbal deficits can be carried out in the usual way, namely by drawing attention to the deficit and its social effect, and by modelling, coaching and rehearsal of more effective behaviour. For homework we suggest that each patient makes a list of his or her deficits on a file card, refers to this before carrying out the daily conversation tasks, and ticks off each deficit that was successfully controlled or corrected, e.g.:

Deficit	Controlled/corrected					
	Mon	Tues	Wed	Thur	Fri	Sat
Mumbling	IIII	IIIII	IIII			
Blank expression	I	I	II			
Looking down	II	III	II			

Face

Two extreme forms of deficit are total facial immobility or with-holding, and over-revealing expression. Between these, particular areas of the face may never be used, such as the eyebrows, or only one or two expressions used, such as neutral and frowning or smiling. Ekman and Friesen (1975) list eight styles or expression habits, the extremes of which can be assumed to be abnormal. In addition to the withholders and revealers mentioned above, there are unwitting expressors, who show emotion without knowing it; blanked expressors, who don't show emotion when they think they do; substitute expressors, who substitute one expression for another without realising it (e.g. feels anger, looks sad); frozen-affect expressors, who show an emotion when in fact they feel neutral (e.g. always looks angry); ever-ready expressors, who show one emotion as a first response to almost any event (e.g. surprise to good news, bad news etc.); and the flooded-affect expressor, who shows one emotion all the time, and this is found in some mental patients.

Another problem commonly found is that expressions – and other non-verbal behaviour – may be knowingly used but the individual has misconceptions about their significance in partic-ular situations.

Smiling is an expression about which there are common mis-conceptions. Patients are usually aware of the display rule which sanctions the social smile in many informal situations, but this may give rise to fixed and continuous smiling, causing mistrust or discomfort in others or giving the impression of submissiveness. Smiling and other expressions should be made more contingent on speech and situational determinants. Some information will be given on this in the section on social routines.

Ekman and Friesen suggest a three-phase exercise to help identify and perhaps control these styles of expression – taking pictures, analysing the pictures, and using a mirror. Some benefit can come from the simpler third phase, summarised as follows: Imitate photographed emotion expressions and check you can do each one in the mirror. Were you successful? Did it feel strange? Imitate the brow-forehead position and look in the mirror. Repeat the above two questions. Repeat the exercise with the other two regions of the face, and repeat the questions. Add the three together and make the total face, and repeat the questions.

Expressions may also be too fleeting, too weak, or 'switched' on and off, and individuals can be trained to express them more quickly, hold them more strongly, for a longer period, and fade them more slowly. Some patients may have a very limited range of expressions, and training should be concentrated on variety.

Voice

A number of exercises can be used to improve production of the vocal elements. For a comprehensive and practical summary of such exercises, see Cole (1964), whose text we follow here.

Resonance. As well as being a 'cue', as in the expression of sadness and warmth, resonance is a basic quality of an attractive speaking voice. It contains five components summed up as FIRM, FREE, FULL FORWARD, FLOWING. *Freedom* can be developed first by humming, being careful that the hum is in the front of the mouth, and then speaking words beginning with M and H. *Firmness* can be practised on explosive consonants, preceded by shut vowels, e.g. oot, ot, ut, at, et, it. *Fullness* involves bringing all the 'resonators' into play, that is the mouth and nasal cavities.

The jaw must be open, free and steady, the tongue kept in light contact with the upper part of the lower teeth as much as possible, while the blade of the tongue does the work. The above tongue position also helps in producing a *forward* sound, for which other tips are: open mouth slowly, trying to imagine you are raising the upper jaw. Alternate the vowels e (wet) and a (ale). A *flowing* quality can be practised by dwelling on the vowel sounds.

Modulation. Pitch should be changed (a) with the emotion expressed, (b) with a change of topic, (c) in speaking an aside.

Inflection. There are six inflections: simple rising, / for continu- ing; simple falling \ for concluding; circumflex rising ∪ for a retorted question; circumflex falling ∩ for emphasis; compound rising ∼ for doubt; and compound falling ⌣ for surprise, viz.:

Is it black or white?

It's blue

Blue?

I think so

Well!

A falling inflection is common among socially inadequate patients and has the effect of concluding a statement and destroying continuity.

Volume. It is often sufficient to point out poor pitch, tone and inflection and model better forms, and patients will make a reasonable change. This is not so for volume, an element which individuals usually find extremely difficult to alter. One method is to use a 'voice key' – a counter operated from an electronic relay which is triggered by a microphone. The key is set off at given volume levels. Rewards are given for counts. It is useful to let an individual take the counter with him and use it at home.

Other non-verbal elements

Attention should be given to the other non-verbal elements listed in the rating scale guide, particularly orientation, posture and gesture. Deficits in these areas are usually self-evident, and cor- rective feedback, instruction and modelling equally straight- forward.

PROBLEMS IN SELF-DISCLOSURE AND FORMALITY

We give below some information and training suggestions for patients who have particular disclosure problems not covered in the subsection above.

Disclosures may vary on a continuum from formal to social, personal to intimate. The training exercises above are aimed at middle range, not too personal disclosures suitable for casual encounters. But patients may need more intensive training to correct problems of under- or over-disclosing, formality or intimacy.

Some patients structure their talk in impersonal and formal ways, avoiding the personal pronoun, emotional expression etc., and also inhibit disclosure about themselves. Buck *et al.* (1974) refer to some individuals as 'internalisers' with high arousal but little expression, and high introversion and sensitivity and low self-esteem. They found evidence that expression of emotion reduces anxiety, inhibition increases it.

The following guide should help to train patients of this kind, i.e. internalisers, to make the content of their talk more informal and personal. (It should be borne in mind that the appropriate level of formality-intimacy varies according to the situation and relationship of the individuals.)

Refer to self in your description. Use 'I' not 'one' or 'it' or 'people in general'.

Use the response frame 'I feel (felt) . . . because . . . ' to begin a statement.

Use more direct emotion words, e.g. '*I* was *quite angry* . . . ', rather than '*It* was *most unfortunate* that . . . '

Practise using face and voice cues simultaneously with emotion words.

Practise making your non-verbal expressions fuller, longer and more intense.

Be more specific and personal in your reference to others and forms of address, e.g. 'Hallo, John', rather than 'Good morning, Mr Smith', and 'John and Fred went', rather than 'The two young gentlemen went'.

Use less of the negative form in expressions: 'It was good', rather than 'It wasn't bad'; 'I'm happy about going', rather than 'I don't mind going'.

Use simple, direct words, rather than long complicated ones. 'I was having a drink', rather than 'I was partaking of refreshment'.

Talk about more personal things i.e. your activities, your home and family, work, interests, etc.

Patients who over-disclose and are too intimate can be guided in the reverse direction, e.g. refer to self less, express fewer and less strong feelings, deintensify non-verbal expression, and avoid talking about personal problems.

NON-VERBAL ACCOMPANIMENTS OF SPEECH

Another area in which therapists may find particular deficits is in the use of kinesic and prosodic markers which accompany speech – to punctuate, emphasise, clarify and colour discourse.

Some of the markers which accompany small verbal units (words, phrases) and which can be modelled and practised include: pausing to think before speaking a new phrase, changing posture before speaking, using head and hand movements, raising pitch and volume on important words and a quick brow raise at the end of a phrase.

Markers accompanying longer units, such as sentences, include: looking up and changing head or arm position.

Longer periods of speech are marked by a gross postural shift involving at least half the body.

Once the basic speaking skills, and any necessary additional training, has been practised, therapist A then summarises the speaker skills section as follows:

'You have all done very well on this section on speaker skills. We have worked mainly on the disclosure of personal information and of feelings. You will find that if you disclose things about yourself, others will disclose more about themselves in return, and will like you more.'

Revision (Exercise 24)

Speakers should now be in a position to give both factual and 'feeling' disclosures, with facial and vocal accompaniments. Now is the time to bring the listener and speaker skills together in a conversation in which both participants can help each other. This is a good exercise for a work triad. After working through the routine in Exercise 24 two or three times (with role-changing and corrective feedback), participants should put their work sheets away and work from memory, making their own spontaneous responses.

This is a convenient session end-point, and Homework Assignment 6 can be given.

References

ARGYLE, M. (1975) *Bodily Communication*. London: Methuen.

BUCK, R., MILLER, R. E. AND CAUL, W. F. (1974) Sex, personality and physiological variables in the communication of affect, via facial expression. *Journal of Personality and Social Psychology*, 30 (4), 587–96.

COLE, W. (1964) *Sound and Sense*. London: Allen & Unwin.

EKMAN, P. AND FRIESEN, W. V. (1975) *Unmasking the Face: A Guide to Recognizing Emotion from Facial Expressions*. New Jersey: Prentice-Hall.

FLOWERS, J. V. AND GUERRA, J. (1974) The use of client coaching in assertion training with large groups. *Community Mental Health Journal*, 10 (4), 414–17.

JOURARD, S. M. (1971) *Self-disclosure: An Experimental Analysis of the Transparent Self*. New York: Wiley.

6. Meshing skills

Briefing

So far, we have kept listener and speaker roles separated, but in normal conversation these roles are blurred by frequent exchanges of the floor, and this involves a further group of activities we have called meshing skills. We have divided these into three areas: (a) content, (b) timing, and (c) turn-taking. We give further exercises in these skills and explain why they are important in maintaining conversations. Content is concerned with the continuity of conversational themes as the floor passes from one participant to the other; timing is concerned with the smooth temporal synchronising of speaking turns and avoidance of synchronies such as simultaneous speech (interruptions) and non-response (delays) (Matarazzo *et al.* 1972); turn-taking is concerned with the cues that signal intentions to start or terminate speaking turns (Duncan 1972).

Presentation

'We have practised some of the skills of listeners and some of the skills of speakers. But normally we do a bit of both, and if we don't do this smoothly, the conversation can break down. For instance, if a new speaker talks about something completely different, which has no connection at all with what the last speaker said, the conversation may become very disjointed and may cause confusion, annoyance or embarrassment. Or if one person does not take up the conversation when it is offered to him, this may be seen as extremely rude and odd. So to keep a conversation flowing smoothly, we need a different set of skills, and that is what we shall now deal with.'

CONTENT (Exercise 25)

'In conversation people talk about similar things – they will have a topic in common. Later they may change the topic. Firstly, then, we shall practise ways of keeping to a common topic. Secondly, we shall practise effective ways of changing a topic.

'You will remember that a speaker message usually includes *factual information, feelings, opinions or beliefs* about a topic. So one thing we can do is to disclose *similar* information and *similar* feelings, opinions and beliefs about a similar topic. Here is an example.' The therapists then demonstrate, e.g.:

Therapist A: 'My car is giving trouble again, and it has only just been serviced. It's infuriating.'

Therapist B: 'I've had a *similar experience*. I had mine serviced two weeks ago, and it wouldn't start this morning. Very annoying.'

This example is compared with the following discontinuous exchange:

Therapist A: 'My car is giving trouble again, and it's only just been serviced. It's infuriating.'

Therapist B: 'The town is so much nicer now they have made all these pedestrian precincts.'

Patients practise this by beginning their disclosures with the words 'I had a similar experience . . . ' or 'The same thing happened to me . . . ' or 'I also . . . ' In this and the following two steps the conversation should be slowed down, so that one speaker can formulate the right responses to the other.

'A second thing we can do is to talk about the same topic but give *different information* or different *feelings* or both.'

> Therapist A: 'I've got a long train journey ahead of me this evening. It's really tedious.'
>
> Therapist B: 'I only have a short bus *journey* but that's *bad* enough.'
> *or*
> 'I also have a long train *journey* but I quite *enjoy* them. It's time to relax and read the newspapers.'
> *or*
> 'I'm travelling by car tonight but I quite enjoy driving.'

'A third thing we can do is to talk about a different topic but keep the *feeling* the same.'

> Therapist A: 'I've got a long train journey ahead of me this evening. It's really tedious.'
>
> Therapist B: 'That may be tedious, but what I find really *bad* is waiting for an hour in the doctor's waiting room.'

'So we have three steps: First, keep topic and feelings the same; second, keep topic the same but change information or feeling; third, keep feeling the same but change the topic.'

Each of these is practised, as given in Exercise 25, and then the three steps are practised as a sequence. Patients will learn that it is better to use steps two or three, since they move the conversation on to new areas.

Therapist A continues: 'After a time, the conversation will move on to a new topic. This may happen gradually through the steps we have just practised. But if you actually want to *change* the topic more abruptly, you must do one of the following: First, wait until there has been a lull in the conversation. Second, interrupt with with an apology and a justification, such as 'I'm sorry but there's something I must tell you.' Third, introduce it as 'by the way'. 'By the way, did you know that . . . ' These three forms are modelled and practised in the normal way.

TIMING (Exercise 26)

Therapist A continues: 'The next thing in running a conversation smoothly is to get the timing right. To get it right, we have to start talking, or make some response, when the other person stops, rather than keep interrupting or lapsing into long silences. Either of these will make the other person cross or feel awkward. I will illustrate what I mean (draws on blackboard):

The normal pattern is: B starts roughly when A stops.	A _____ B _____
It's usually wrong to keep talking at the same time as the other	A _____ B _____
It's also usually wrong to leave a long silence before responding to A.	A _____ B ____

Therapist B begins a demonstration conversation and therapist A responds in each of these ways in turn, with therapist B showing his discomfort after the asynchronous responses. After a second demonstration, therapist B is asked to verbalise these feelings (Exercise 26). Patients then practise timing.

One patient is encouraged to reward his partner for good timing by immediately responding with further disclosures and being friendly, and to 'punish' poor responses by remaining silent for a time (15 seconds). The partner is asked in turn to reward the first patient for good disclosures by an immediate listener response or disclosure of his own. In this way both patients mutually reinforce each other. The monitor keeps a record of the partner's right or wrong responses, or ideally records the interaction on an event recorder, which gives visual feedback in the form shown in the above diagram. Alternatively, another patient or one of the therapists can give each partner contingent reinforcement for correct responses from the observation room via an ear microphone. The emphasis in this exercise, as in other parts of training, is to get the patient to experience the effect of his behaviour on the other.

TURN-TAKING (Exercises 27, 28)

Therapist A continues: 'Some people find it difficult to get the timing right because they don't know *when* to respond or start speaking, or even when to stop speaking. How do people tell each other *when* they want a response, *when* they want the other to take up the conversation and *when* they want to take it up again? In this exercise we shall practise the techniques for doing all these things.'

Below and after Exercise 29 we list a number of turn-taking cues under five headings, each with a description of its function and the intended message. The therapists should demonstrate each in turn, alternating speaker role as appropriate. Patients practise after each demonstration (Exercises 27, 28). Finally, the whole series is practised as a sequence, with one participant initiating the sequence, i.e. speaks, hands over, takes up, maintains, suppresses turn claim, hands over, resists hand-over.

Handing-over – meaning: 'I have finished what I wanted to say. Over to you.'

(i) Ask the other a question and continue looking at him. This may include leaning forward. The question should follow up your own disclosure, such as 'What did you think?' 'Do you find that?' 'Do you agree?' Or you can use a questioning statement like, 'I don't know what you think'.

(ii) As you reach the end of a period of talking look at the other, finish your verbal message, then look away. If you have been gesturing, return hands to rest as you stop talking. Lower the pitch of your voice (downward inflection) on your last word or two. Optional: use a concluding phrase like 'So that's it' or 'You-know'. Don't start a new phrase, or use a conjunction like 'and' or 'but', as this is a cue that you want to continue. In other words, conclude on a complete phrase.

Taking-up – meaning: 'Finish what you want to say. I want to take up the conversation.'

Some of the following are for extreme cases, where the other person is reluctant to stop.

(iii) Prepare the other that you are going to take up the conversation by: Rapid head-nods or shakes; rapid repetition of 'yes', 'mhmm', or 'no'; by leaning forward and/or making several major body shifts.

(iv) Withhold any response until the others stops speaking. Then take up the conversation.

(v) Use a simple reflection, picking up a word or phrase, but then keep the floor by continuing with your own disclosure.

(vi) Begin strongly, with fairly loud voice, clear enunciation, pitch different from the other's, avoidance of speech errors, such as repetitions ('I-I thought . . .'). Finally, *keep talking* until after the other gives up the conversation before you pause.

(vii) In groups, get the talker's attention (orienting reflex) by major body shifts, body and face orientation and listener responses such as (v). Take up the conversation immediately the talker responds to you.

(viii) Interrupt the other during a pause for thought (e.g. when he says 'ummm' or 'err'), or at the end of a clause/phrase of speech.

Suppressing a turn claim – meaning: 'I'd like to carry on. I'm not letting you take over.'

(ix) As you reach your point, don't pause, don't look at the other, continue gesturing, talk louder.

Resisting a hand-over – meaning: 'I don't want to take over. You carry on.'

(x) Use a listener response and keep looking at the other, e.g. head-nod, reflection, 'mhmm-mhmm'.

(xi) Ask a question, or turn the other's question around, viz: 'I'm not sure, what do you think?' 'First I'd like to hear more of what you think. Do you . . . ?' Then continue looking at the other.

Continuing – meaning: 'May I carry on? Give me more feedback.'

(xii) As you reach the end of a clause look at the other, then look away and continue talking and gesturing.

(xiii) In addition to looking at other, and making your point, ask for feedback, viz: 'Don't you think?', then continue talking.

References

DUNCAN, S. (1972) Some signals and rules for taking speaking turns in conversations. *Journal of Personality and Social Psychology*, 23, 283–92

MATARAZZO, J. D. AND WIENS, A. N. (1972) *The Interview: Research on its Anatomy and Structure*. Chicago Ill.: Aldine Atherton.

7. Expression of attitudes

Briefing

In the previous sections we have dealt mainly with one level of interpersonal communication – the part that forms social conversation. We shall now deal more fully with another level – the attitude expressed to the person sharing the conversation. We shall revise the two main interpersonal attitudes and explain their importance, function and behavioural elements, and give some exercises in expressing these attitudes.

Presentation

'In this session we shall learn how to express friendliness and assertiveness while we speak and listen. But first, let's revise an earlier part of the programme. People do two things in conversation. Firstly, they talk about their experience and feelings – and we have practised that. Secondly, and at the same time, people express feelings and attitudes to each other, such as friendliness, dominance, aggressiveness and so on. The first is what people *talk* about and it's out in the open and we can reflect back and so on. The second is what people do – they *adopt* or *have* attitudes to each other, but *don't* usually talk about them (except in very close relationships). So while we can reflect back people's emotions (because it's something they tell us) we don't reflect back their attitude in the same way. Instead, we use that information in another way – to help us choose another attitude in return. If Fred adopts a superior attitude to me, what attitude or style do I adopt? We have already dealt with the main attitudes and the recognition of their elements. We now turn to the selection and performance of these.

'You will remember that there are two important attitudes or styles: There is friendliness as against unfriendliness, and assertiveness as against submissiveness.' The behaviour which comprises these attitudes was given in Exercise 10.

CHOOSING A STYLE (Exercise 29)
'In the next exercise we should bear in mind that whenever we interact with others, we have to do two things in addition to listening and speaking about topics and events. We have to

observe the other person's attitude to us and we have to *choose* a style or attitude which is either *similar to* or *different from* the other's. Thus, if we observe the other is cold, we can choose to be cold, or we can choose some other style – dominance, warmth, etc. So the next exercise (29) will take the form of a conversation in which one person's task is to combine speaker skills with attitude expression; in other words, he will talk about some topic in a friendly or unfriendly, a dominant or a submissive way. The second person's task is to observe the other's attitudes and the content of his talk, to choose a style *and* a topic in response, and to perform *both* of these.'

The therapists then demonstrate this, verbalising their observations and choices, e.g.:

Therapist A: 'First, I'll choose a style – I'll be friendly and informal to B. Second, I'll choose a topic: I'll talk about Christmas shopping. Here goes (leans towards B, smiles etc.). "I've just started my Christmas shopping, and I've never seen such crowds and queues . . . ".'

Therapist B: 'First, I'll identify his attitude and what he's talking about. He seems friendly and he's talking about Christmas shopping. Second, I'll choose my style and what to talk about in return – I'll be friendly, too, and tell him I've started Christmas shopping too, and how bad the parking is . . . Here goes.' B then carries out his intentions.

CHOOSING FOR EFFECT (Exercise 30)

After Exercise 29, therapist A continues: 'The next thing we must remember is that the style of behaviour of one person will affect the style of the other. If you are cold, the other person will probably be cold in response. If you are warm, the other is likely to be warm. If you are assertive, the other may respond by being assertive or submissive, depending on him and the situation. People choose their style *in order to* affect each other's behaviour in this way. So, when we choose a style, we have to ask "How does he want to affect me?" "How do I want to affect him?"'

Therapists demonstrate and patients practice Exercise 30.

It is difficult to suggest ideal response styles because these depend so much on situations and on particular patients' deficits. We have found that the commonest deficits are coldness and submissiveness, and therefore suggest that the following styles should be practised most:

In general: More warmth and more assertiveness
In particular interactions:
Respond to warmth with warmth

Respond to coldness with warmth first, then assertiveness with warmth.

Respond to assertiveness with assertiveness.

Respond to submissiveness with warmth.

Revision (Exercise 31)

To finally round off all the training so far, patients are guided through a complete conversation routine, from greeting to parting. Exercise 31 is one way of revising this

References

GRANT, E. C. (1968) An ethological description of non-verbal behaviour during interviews. *British Journal of Medical Psychology*, 41, 177–84.

GRANT, E. C. (1971) Facial expressions and gesture. *Journal of Psychosomatic Research*, 15, 391–4.

MEHRABIAN, A. (1972) *Nonverbal Communication*. Chicago, Ill.: Aldine Atherton.

SCHEFLEN, A. E. AND SCHEFLEN, A. (1972) *Body Language and the Social Order*. New Jersey: Prentice-Hall.

8. Social routines

So far we have dealt with what might be called the basic conversation skills. We now come to a group of behavioral routines, of which greetings and partings are one kind, which are different in structure and function from those dealt with so far in that they are more standardised, have symbolic rather than literal meaning, and serve to initiate, terminate, confirm, restore and change social interaction. These routines, discussed briefly in the assessment chapter, have been likened to rituals and ceremonies in that the words and actions are bound by strict procedural rules, are widely recognised in a culture, and, most importantly, are obligatory in certain situations. Training in these routines is important, not because patients are necessarily unaware of them, but rather because they may fail to *use* them or to recognise the consequences of this lack of use. Failure to use such routines often results in giving offence or insult and in possible rejection. All routines are actions performed in a given sequence, but there is a variety of forms due to cultural variations. We give examples of some of the commonest forms, drawing where possible on well substantiated findings but otherwise on experience and observation, but attention should be paid to the culture, class, age, sex, status and relationships of the individual concerned.

We have grouped routines into five kinds: greetings and partings; routines for initiating and changing situations; remedies (apologies and accounts); routines for confirming, supporting and giving; and routines for asserting rights and refusing. This is suggested as a practical classification and does not necessarily accord with theoretical considerations (e.g. Goffman 1972).

The analysis of routines is rather complex, but it is neither necessary nor desirable to impart much of this information to patients. A better policy is to get patients to try out the basic exercise routines, and the therapists to correct and inform them when necessary. We give below a blow-by-blow behavioural description of the main social routines for therapists' background information, while patients follow the simplified practice, Exercises 32–46.*

Greetings and partings

This section is concerned with greeting and parting routines, or what Goffman (from whom we draw) calls 'ritual brackets surrounding periods of heightened access'. Two greetings and a 'non-greeting' (or 'civil inattention') are described, also a standard parting sequence.

Greetings combine a demonstration of friendly intention with a request for social interaction in a way that other verbal devices,

* It should be noted at this point that general homework assignments have been discontinued in the Trainee's Handbook, and it is left to therapists to construct appropriate assignments. These should now be stepped up to include more ambitious social initiatives around social themes such as joining a club, holding a party, inviting someone out, offering help and so on.

such as questions, do not. For this reason, they are usually obligatory as forms of address. Moves in a greeting sequence also require
responses in the same way that questions require answers. Thus
the greeter places the other under an obligation to respond in a
fairly specific way. In the behavioural descriptions that follow we
refer to responses which satisfy this rule as *reciprocal*, and ones
which break it and which disrupt interaction, cause offence and
so on, as *unreciprocal*. So long as these basic rules of address and
reciprocity are satisfied, interactors have the option, at any stage
of a greeting, of continuing or terminating the interaction, without
giving offence or losing face. This option is lost once the greeting
ends and conversation begins, and an entirely different routine – a
parting – must then be used to terminate the interaction. The term
open is used to refer to moves which request or invite further
interaction, and *closed* to refer to acts which terminate interaction.

INTERACTION GREETING (Exercise 32)

First move:

> *Sighting.* Observation and identification of other by glance
> or over-hearing, and decision to greet. The decision
> depends on need or desire to meet other, urgency of
> need, other's attitude, what other is doing at the time.
> *Distant salutation*: Face-to-face orientation and mutual
> glance, followed by eyebrow flash, smile, open-palm
> greeting gesture, brief verbal greeting with head toss, etc.
> *Function :* Initiate social contact with further interaction
> open (e.g. 'I want to be on friendly terms and I am open
> for a brief chat, are you?').

Response:

> The response may be reciprocal and open (i.e. the
> same as above), completing the first sequence and lead-
> ing to the second; or closed, such as a parting greeting
> terminating the interaction. An unreciprocal act would
> be a 'non-greeting' breaking a social rule and would
> constitute an 'affront'.

Second move:

> *Approach and preparation :* Gaze cut off, head dipped,
> ongoing activity stopped, and approach to other begun.
> *Final approach :* Mutual gaze, smiling, head tilted,
> palm presented.

Close salutation: Halt and take up face-to-face position, hand shake or other body contact (sometimes), verbal greeting and conventional questions ('How are you?'). Function: This is an open move to consolidate social contact and seek extended interaction ('Given that we are on friendly terms, I'd like to have a conversation with you. Are you agreeable?'). (Note: As well as saying 'I care about you', the conventional question 'How are you?' is sometimes asking: 'Are you agreeable to chat?')

Response:

Again, the response may be reciprocal and open (equivalent non-verbal behaviour and the verbally conventional: 'Fine, and you?') resulting in a third move; or closed (a parting routine); or it may be non-reciprocal (treated as a variant of the passing greeting or more commonly, leave-taking) ending the interaction. A passing greeting here would also be an 'affront'.

Third move:

Attachment phase: Move to take up a position for an extended conversation, non-verbally maintaining an open, friendly, interpersonal attitude. He will use a verbal comment (usually an implied question) referring to the context that justifies the greeter's waylaying the other for conversation, for example: 'Haven't seen you for ages', or 'Fancy seeing you here', or 'Thanks for the drink the other night'. We call this a bridging phrase, connecting the greeter in some way with the other's world. This is followed by 'basic conversation', e.g. questions etc.
Function: An open move which further consolidates interaction into true (not conventionalised) conversation. Example of use: To make new friends or celebrate meeting old ones.

Response:

This again may be reciprocated or the other may end the interaction with closed sequence such as a parting.

Fourth move:

The greeter may at this stage choose a closing move such as a parting (see below).

This shows that each person can keep the interaction open or closed at any point by use of an acceptable convention.

PASSING GREETING (Exercise 33)

Elements: Some of the following – face-to-face orientation, eye contact, raising of eyebrows (eyebrow 'flash'), cheek 'flick' or smiling, small hand gesture, head nod, brief verbal greeting ('hi'). These occur simultaneously, are muted and terminated after one or two seconds with a look away and ahead if walking (i.e. a closed act).

Function: Recognition only, i.e. a closed move to maintain social contact without interacting (e.g. 'I consider we are acquaintances but don't want to stop and talk').

Example of use: Passing by acquaintances on daily routine as at work. A reciprocal closed response completes this sequence.

'NON-GREETING' (Exercise 34)

Elements: Face-to-face orientation; 'dead-eyeing' (i.e. brief mutual glance followed by downward gaze shift). All other behaviour: no change (i.e. does not stop ongoing activity).

Function: A closed move to signal mutual respect and lack of fear, but no social contact intended.

Example of use: in the street, buses, tubes, and other public places when face to face with strangers. Also with famous people, crippled and handicapped people. A reciprocal closed response completes this sequence. *Not* used with acquaintances except when passing on several occasions in a single day.

PARTINGS (Exercise 35)

Partings bring the interaction to a definite close, sum up the consequences of the encounter for the relationship, and bolster the relationship for the anticipated period of no contact. Like greetings, partings may have several moves, more complex ones tending to follow the longer greetings. It will be seen that the order of moves is to some extent a mirror image of the interaction greeting.

First move:

> Breaks postural frame, e.g. steps back, looks down and away, turns out from other; kinesic signals of departure; verbal comment justifying leaving at that point, e.g. 'Is that clock right? I'll get the sack.', '. . . . ,The wife will murder me'.
>
> *Function:* To reassure the other, e.g. 'I am not leaving because I want to, but because I have to'.

Response:

> A reciprocal closing response may give a similar reason for having to depart ('I, too, have to leave') or simply reassure the leaver that his justification is acceptable, leading to the second move. A unreciprocal move may take the form of the other ignoring the leaver's first sequence and carrying on with the interaction. Both resist closing the interaction. A reciprocal closing response leads to:

Second move:

> Takes up position for departure, e.g. if seated, stands up; initiates 'parting' – looks at other, smiling, possibly shakes hands, touches shoulder, etc., gives conventional verbal 'respects' (e.g. 'Nice to see you again.' 'Hope we meet again soon.' 'We will have to arrange something . . . keep in touch.').
>
> *Function:* To bolster relationship for period of no contact.

Response:

> The other may reciprocate closing in like manner, leading to third move, or resist by verbal insistence on continuing, with reference to some justification ('You can't be in that much of a hurry').

Third move:

> Eye contact, smile, face-to-face orientation but body orientation away from other; walking away, farewell gesture, verbal parting and use of other's name ('Bye, John'). This display lasts only two or three seconds and

is terminated by breaking gaze with turn of the head and termination of gesture.

Function : Definite termination.

Example of use of above parting : After extended period of talk with a friend, or person in superior position, particularly in anticipation of period of separation.

Response:

Again, the other may close with a simultaneous farewell, or resist closing with a verbal postscript. This latter is a useful device for adding something without affecting the sequential order of the farewell or necessitating a new one. A disruptive 'rule-breaking' non-reciprocation would be an open question such as 'er . . . . How's the wife after her operation?'

As with greetings there are conventions for stopping and starting the parting sequence. Rule-breaking responses occur when one of the interactors does not follow the proper sequence, as in the above example.

A full parting is only needed if the interactors have paused or stopped to talk or if there is likely to be a period of separation. If the interactor does not pause – as in the passing greeting – no parting is needed and would be considered out of place if used. Similarly, if the interactors are likely to meet frequently during the day, an attenuated parting only would be appropriate. In addition, the full three-move parting is only used after a period of original (non-ritual) conversation. For instance, if used immediately after the second or third greeting sequence, then the greeter would only use the first and third moves of the parting:

1st   A: Have to rush

       B: Sure

3rd   A: See you

       B: O.K.

Presentation

'So far, we have been working mainly on the skills involved after a conversation is underway. Now we will concentrate on ways of starting conversations – or any kind of interaction. In most situations we don't just start talking to someone out of the blue. We don't start talking unless invited to do so, and we don't get invited unless we ask – in some way – for 'permission' in the first place. Fortunately, we have a convenient convention, namely a greeting, which does all this for us.'

Patients are introduced to the three kinds of greeting routines and the parting routine, and the moves described. Demonstrations are given and patients follow the moves from the exercises. During the exercises, rather than practise each move bit by bit, it is better to get patients to try out a complete practice routine, participants using the full length of the room while being monitored. This is followed by corrective feedback on elements or moves missed out, including background information when necessary, and finally by rehearsal of a better sequence. The negative consequences of leaving out obligatory greeting moves and responses are emphasised. After the moves and elements have been reasonably learned, role-play simulations of actual and possible problem situations should be noted and practised.

Initiating and changing

Another group of social responses have the main function of initiating and changing interactions. The importance is self-evident, in that failure to use them greatly limits the capacity of an individual to bring about change in his social environment. Some of these routines have already been dealt with, namely questions and greetings. We are concerned here with those routines which call for specific interpersonal action on the part of the other, namely requests, commands and demands. The request is the most common and is also the weaker form in that, being a question, it offers a choice of compliance or refusal. However, the request makes either compliance or refusal obligatory and has considerable force in affecting the behaviour of others. In this section we deal with (i) requests per se and (ii) gaining access, i.e. the use of greetings, questions and requests in gaining access to strangers in different settings.

REQUESTS (Exercise 36)

Requests are appropriate in situations where a person has limited or no rights in carrying out some action himself, or in asking others to carry out an action, but must nonetheless be justifiable and reasonable in terms of the relationship and the situation. As well as asking permission for a specific action to be performed, a request implies recognition and respect for the other's rights. Failure to make a request and making demands would in this situation be a transgression of rights and would be regarded as a personal slight. In some situations, therefore, requests are obligatory, but can be made in a form which makes refusal very difficult.

Training should be given by supplying or eliciting examples of request-making, and asking the initial question: 'Is this request reasonable?' Perfunctory requests such as asking the time or for a light can be made in most situations and most kinds of relationship, but more serious and personal requests need to be justified by the strength of the relationship (friends not strangers) and/or the situation. If the request is reasonable, the request routine begins as follows:

First move:

> *Request:* Give non-verbal 'immediacy' cues; make verbal request of the form 'Can I . . . please?' or 'Will you . . . please?' stated directly and to the point, or in the case of more serious or less justifiable forms, preceded by a preparatory statement such as 'I hope you won't mind me asking but . . . ', 'The reason I rang/came over was . . . ', 'I'm in a bit of a fix . . . '
>
> *Function:* Show respect, optimise compliance.

Response:

> A *compliant* response includes a verbal agreement to allow the request and an expression of willingness, which may vary from reluctance to enthusiasm, and is conveyed non-verbally (e.g. annoyance or happiness), verbally (e.g. 'I suppose so' or 'You're very welcome/with pleasure'). A *refusal* includes a verbal statement disallowing the request, and an expression of varying degrees of remorse, with appropriate non-verbal accompaniments (e.g. 'Certainly not' or 'I'm terribly sorry but I can't because . . . ').

Second move:

> *Appreciation:* The second move to the compliant response continues with non-verbal immediacy cues plus smiling and an appreciative gesture, and verbally with an expression of gratitude and possibly a reason

(e.g. 'Thank you very much. You have helped me out of a fix'). The second move to a refusal can take a number of forms, including appreciation and acceptance of the excuse ('Thanks anyway'), pressing the request further ('Oh come on'), seeking justification for the refusal ('Surely you can't mean it?').

Response:

The successful request sequence – request, compliance, appreciation – may end with a *minimisation* response ('It's O.K.' 'It's nothing') or simply a small gesture. An unsuccessful request sequence may end with a brief apology.

After practising the main request routine, various modifications to fit supplied situations should be worked out. This should begin with the situation suggested in Exercise 37, modelled by the therapists. In this situation A wants to make a personal request of B, who is a stranger, so the routine is modified as follows:

A	*B*
First: greeting/introduction	Ditto
Second: extended conversation(s)	Ditto
Third: request	Compliance or refusal
Fourth: appreciation	Minimisation or apology

Some examples of role-playing could include: A asks B to lend him some money; A asks B, a stranger, to do something for him.

Presentation

The first therapist introduces the idea of requests and their importance in bringing about change in the social environment, e.g. 'Most people feel inhibited about asking certain things of others, like borrowing something, asking a favour or a date, for fear of giving offence or being turned down. This causes some to hold back, to withdraw, feel frustrated and ineffective and possibly depressed. We shall deal with some techniques for overcoming this problem, the first being *making requests*.'

He also explains their function and describes the steps and choices in a request routine. The therapists then demonstrate the request routine and the example in Exercise 36. Patients role-play the same example, and try examples of their own, or situations supplied by the therapists.

GAINING ACCESS TO STRANGERS

We have now discussed the main routines for overtly initiating and changing interaction, namely greetings, questions and requests. It should be pointed out that other routines, such as confirming, supporting, giving and apologising, can also be used, though in a less obvious way. In this section, we will discuss one important application of initiating routines – gaining access to strangers in various settings. This is not only a major problem with socially inadequate patients, but an essential skill for people with a restricted social life.

Starting interactions with strangers consists of two consecutive parts – access conventions or 'ice-breakers', followed by the exchange of identities, such as occupation, place of living etc.

There are at least three types of situations where strangers may meet, each with their own access conventions, which we have divided as follows: private social situations; public situations structured for meeting strangers, and public situations not so structured (this classification is made on practical, not theoretical, grounds).

Private social situations, such as a club or private party, are settings where members have a common bond and are bound by rules of conduct. A general point about private situations is that strangers have much greater access to each other where there is a common bond and members have the security of knowing that newcomers will be vetted and can be expected to behave reasonably. There is therefore less need for strangers to justify their mutual advances.

Public situations structured for meeting strangers include dance halls and discos, where there are clear 'access' conventions but equally clear protective techniques, and much risk of refusal and loss of face. This would be a very advanced task for male patients, and careful preparation is required. In most cases it would be inadvisable to suggest this task, and we do not include a suggested routine.

Finally, there are situations which are not specially structured for meeting strangers, but nonetheless have clear access conventions for so doing, such as in the street, in launderettes, pubs, cafes, etc.

Presentation.
The patients are introduced as follows: 'We have worked on greetings, which will help you to get to know acquaintances better. In this section, we will work on ways of starting conversations with strangers. We will take two types of situations where strangers meet, and work through some techniques for "breaking the ice" and getting acquainted.'

Private social situations (Exercise 37)
A club will be taken as an example. Here are some of the appropriate conventions both for 'breaking the ice' and exchanging identities.

'Breaking the ice'.   Introduction by a third party: a common friend or official of the club introduces the two individuals. A new member will usually benefit from this convention, but must get to know one individual fairly well (it is usually easier to start with a club official).

Self-introduction: This type of greeting is common in a form such as the following: Initial greeting; conventional aside or request for information; introduction of self; justifying account for the introduction.

'Priming' an acquaintance to introduce him to a stranger he knows. This is preferably done implicitly, by use of 'immediacy' cues such as proximity, looking expectantly at acquaintance; or explicitly, by asking to be introduced.

Request to join ongoing activity, and use of implicit spatial cues as above.

Setting the situation up. For example, giving yourself a social function such as taking around the drink tray.

This is probably the optimal situation for patients, simply because access is fairly easy and the technique fairly straightforward, involving less danger of loss of face compared with the situations described below.

Exchange of identities.   If 'ice-breaking' is successful, the two strangers will proceed to exchange information about identities. Some of this information will already be conveyed by physical appearance, and patients should be conscious of the messages they are sending by their clothes, hair (including beard) and cosmetics, about their age, social class, social group and status.

Information disclosed or requested will be about place of living, occupation and work status, possessions, achievements, member- ship of groups or organisations and social connections, marital status and parenthood, and so on.

Public situations (Exercise 38)
Examples are: in the street, launderettes, libraries, pubs and coffee bars. The sequence here is 'breaking the ice', following-up and exchanging identities.

'Breaking the ice'.   Requests or offers of the following kind: information (e.g. direction to a place, hours of opening, prices of various things etc.), or advice (e.g. how to operate a launderette machine, a one-armed bandit in a pub etc.), or a favour (asking for a light, the time, to sit in the vacant seat, etc.).

Conventional asides of the following kind: comment about the general situation (e.g. the weather), and the specific situation (e.g. the bus service or other service being used at the time, or whatever is happening at the moment).

Following up.   This can be about: the topic introduced (e.g. after 'Nice weather' 'Wonder how long it'll last?' 'Surprising for the time of year . . . ' etc.) 'This' place (e.g. 'Is this a new pub?' 'What's the beer like?' 'The service seems slow').

The people 'here' (e.g. 'Crowded tonight', 'Noisy place'). Other's connection with this place ('Is this your local?' 'Are you a visitor?').

This is followed by the exchange of identities, much as in the previous section.

Confirming, supporting and giving

Another group of social routines has the function of confirming and supporting relationships, either symbolically, with compli- ments, praise, congratulations, encouragement and sympathy, or tangible, with gifts, loans or actions. These routines, like greetings, are obligatory in some situations, since failure to use them would give offence. When not obligatory, their use is still important, since they are powerful techniques for strengthening bonds and making friendships.

OFFERING COMPLIMENTS, PRAISE, CONGRATULATIONS, ENCOURAGEMENT, SYMPATHY (Exercise 39)

We suggest that compliments are used mainly for such tangible everyday things as aspects of the other's self-presentation – clothes, hairstyle, jewellery, slimness etc. – and for the quality of their entertainment, such as food and wine, and so on. Praise is used for less tangible achievements, such as creativity, enterprise and sacrifice, while congratulations are used for achievements completed, e.g. a qualification, award, promotion or changed personal status such as engagement, marriage or parenthood. These, as well as encouragement and sympathy, seem to follow a fairly common routine.

First move:
> Non-verbal 'immediacy' cues (mutual glance, direct orientation, possible physical contact, such as a handshake, hand on arm); expression of appropriate emotion (pleasure, sadness); conventional verbal expression of compliment, encouragement, etc. and reference to reason for this.
> *Function:* Affirmation or support.

Response:
> The response will contain two parts: verbal expression of thanks and appreciation with reciprocation of non-verbal warmth; expression of appropriate affect, which would include modesty for achievements, happiness for change in personal status, sadness for personal loss. This will sometimes end the sequence, or:

Second move:
> Question about the circumstances, followed by a listener routine.

Response:
> The responder would give an account of the circumstances and experiences associated with it.

OFFERING TO GIVE, LEND AND DO THINGS (Exercise 40)

A similar behavioural routine applies to offering to give, lend and do more tangible things, and is also an important part of strengthening friendship bonds. The kinds of things given or actions offered are also bound by conventions – of familiarity or appropriateness. Newly acquainted individuals, such as patients in the group, may begin by doing or lending small, useful things, going on to give items made by themselves or to do things which have more affiliative significance. The verbal elements of a given routine would include:

First move:

   The offer, and a reference to the reason for making it.

Response:

   A response combining thanks and reassurance about the offer.

Second move:

   Confirmation of the offer, possible insistence upon acceptance.

Response:

   A response of acceptance, thanks and confirmation of the appropriateness of the offer: or a refusal, thanks and face-saving reason for refusal (to be dealt with in more detail later.)

Third move:

   Minimisation of sacrifice and a possible emphasis on the pleasure of giving.

Remedies

Almost any socially adventurous or assertive act risks causing a slight or some offence and a consequent rejection or rebuke, and the anticipatory fear of this causes many socially inadequate or phobic patients to avoid the use of such initiatives. The social routines so far described have built-in safeguards, but often these are not enough.

   This section deals with those conventions and rituals which Goffman calls remedial interchanges and which skilled people use to remedy the offence, to make their actions acceptable, and thereby reduce the likelihood of the actor being anxious when he asserts himself. A patient may use the remedial skills badly, or fail to use them at all; this may result in resentment on the part of the other, which the patient then interprets as personal dislike. Alternatively, a patient may over-use them, e.g. in making an abject apology, resulting in loss of face and self-esteem.

Presentation

'When we take some social initiative as would follow from the previous exercises, there is always a risk we'll upset someone, or get rejected or rebuffed, usually inadvertently. We shall discuss three techniques for remedying the situation – giving accounts of our action (explaining or excusing it), apologising, and, in the last resort, saving face.

ACCOUNTS (Exercise 41)

An account denies, explains or excuses our act in at least four ways, ranging from full to partial diminution of blame.

A denial that the act was performed, e.g. 'I did not do it/had nothing to do with it'.

Explanation that the act was misinterpreted: 'It did not happen that way.'

Explanation that the act was done in all innocence: 'I did not realise . . . '

Explanation that the act was done under circumstances of reduced responsibility. 'I could not help myself.'

The last two accounts would be accompanied by an apology, the first should never be, and the second might be, depending on the situation.

APOLOGIES (Exercise 42)

An apology accepts at least partial blame and has some or all of the following elements (Goffman 1972): 'Expression of embarrassment and chagrin; clarification that one knows what conduct has been expected and sympathises with the application of negative sanction; verbal rejection, repudiation and disavowal of the wrong way of behaving along with vilification of the self that so behaved; espousal of the right ways and an avowal henceforth to pursue that course; performance of penance and the volunteering of restitution.'

The following is a suggested apology routine with some of the possible alternative moves, including accounts.

First move:

    (a) The *apology*: non-verbal immediacy cues, serious or sad expression; vocally expressive with variable pitch and medium volume; verbal apology with use of word 'sorry' or 'apologise', depending on formality of situation.

    (b) Acknowledgement of *rule-breaking*.

    (c) Possible *reflection* of other's discomfort, and feelings towards apologiser.

    (d) Offer of *account* minimising blame.

    (e) *Self-disclosure* of feelings of embarrassment, guilt, shame.

    (f) Possible acceptance of *punishment*.

    (g) *Promise* of future good behaviour.

    (h) Terminates apology, stops talking, looks back at other, changes and relaxes posture, terminates gesture etc., i.e. hands conversation over.

Response:

Other gives *relief* ('Never mind') or *demands account* ('Why did you do it?'), whether already given or not, or questions apologiser on any of the components (a) to (g) which leads to re-run of the apology sequence. However, instead of returning to the first move, apologiser moves to the second.

Second move:

Repeats first move in attenuated form, then terminates apology with words such as 'That's really *all* I can say', and immediately changes the conversation, using, if necessary, takeover suppression signals.

Function: Request that apology sequence be concluded.

Response:

Other gives relief and gives reply to new topic, ending this move and the apology routine.

Alternatively, he may still demand a further account: 'Before we go on to that I still want to know . . . ' or further questions the apologiser.

Optional third move:

> Repeats first sequence as an overt repetition, i.e. 'I have apologised, I have given an explanation, etc. . . . ', then
>
> Makes termination of apology overt with assertive behaviour – eye contact, face-to-face orientation, frowning, high tonus, forward lean, loud voice, emphatic gestures.
>
> Verbal: 'That's an end to it, I don't intend to say anything more about it. O.K.?'
>
> *Function*: Each step makes it more difficult to make covert demands of further apology. The third sequence demands that apology sequence be concluded.

Response:

> Acquiescence and relief ends the sequence. Further demands may be made, but here the interchange has escalated to a confrontation, a step the other would normally be reluctant to take.

SAVING FACE (Exercise 43)

Saving face means minimising the embarrassment and consequent anxiety an individual may feel after he has exposed himself in some way to rebuke or rejection such as making a request or making a 'faux pas' or some other social 'accident'. This is a large area, and we will have to confine ourselves to general comment and one kind of situation – handling rebuffs. Patients report that learning to cope skilfully with such situations makes them less anxious and less likely to withdraw from other social situations where a similar accident might occur.

The problem about rebuffs of the rule-following kind (i.e. where the other offers a face-saving formula) is their ambiguity. Is the excuse genuine, or is this truly a polite rebuff? The following suggestion aims to cover the problem; it is of a similar form to the request sentence:

First move and response:

> Greeting/Introduction.

Second move and response:

> Hold extended conversation.

Third move:

> Make the request (e.g. asking for a date) with accompanying warm attitude.

Response:
>
> Refusal with excuse (possibly face-saving) (e.g. 'Sorry, but I'm washing my hair').

Fourth move:
>
> A second request is made (e.g. 'Well, how about Saturday, then?').

Response:
>
> The request is turned down with another (face-saving) account.

Fifth move:
>
> This move is directed to the explicit, conventional message (i.e. the hair washing) *not* to the implicit message (which may or may not be 'I don't really want to go out with you'). The move contains acceptance of the explicit reason, and a non-specific invitation giving reassurance that the requester has not lost face and that no damage has been done to the relationship (e.g. 'Never mind, we'll have to arrange another date').

Response:
>
> Acceptance of the 'invitation' (e.g. 'Yes O.K.'). This may be a conventional response, recognising that the invitation has a more symbolic than literal meaning, and often carries an additional meaning like 'Thanks for not making me feel guilty'.

Sixth move:
>
> This is an optional move which converts the second move from a ritual to a substantive invitation, i.e. the invitation is made explicit ('I really mean it. I'll give you a ring'). This leaves the situation open, with the invitation having been made but the responder not obliged to comply or refuse. The interaction thus ends on a constructive and possibly hopeful note.

Face-saving sequences lend themselves well to modelling and role-playing, though they make 'advanced' homework assignments.

Assertive routines

We have described some of the social routines for initiating and changing the behaviour of others, and some ways of remedying slights and offences which these actions inevitably incur. The reverse situation is now introduced, where the other initiates and the patient is the potentially offended party and his self-esteem is at risk. There are a number of common routines for protecting one's rights, such as refusing, demanding apologies and redress, resisting and reversing 'put-downs' and saving face generally. We use the term 'assertion' to mean this kind of activity, which is a more restricted use of the term than is customary.

Presentation

'So far, we have dealt with the role of the offender. Now we will work on the role of the person offended. The main question here is: If the other violates your rights – jumps ahead of you in a queue, keeps interrupting in conversation, fails to give you the service you asked and paid for, makes unreasonable demands on you, etc. – what is the most skilled way of asserting your right?'

ASSERTION (Exercise 44)

Patients are asked to imagine or recall a situation in which they think they should *assert or have asserted their rights* and to ask the following question: 'Is the other really transgressing my rights?' How sure am I that the offender could not fully or partly excuse his action, e.g. where it was an accident, a mistake, done in ignorance, done in my best interest? etc.'

In the following, one example is taken for simplicity, where B persists in transgressing the rights of A and the remedy includes not only an apology but a restoration of 'substance' (involving the return of something or the reversal of an action). A situation is chosen, preferably a patient's, where the outcome is ambiguous – the question of rights, of excusability, is at the start an open one, e.g. 'You are in a crowded grocery store and in a hurry. You pick one small item and get in line to pay for it. You are really trying to hurry because you're already late for an appointment. Then, a woman with a shopping cart full of groceries cuts in line in front of you.'

The answer to the initial question is that this is an apparent transgression, but a justifying account or excuse is possible, such as (a) it's new stock for the other side of the shop, (b) it has already been paid for and this is the quickest exit, etc.

First move:

> This move is a cautious one because there is some uncertainty about justifying reasons. It takes the form of an implicit request. The first step, then, is to 'prime' the offender by pointing out the apparent offence – a ritual move recognised by most people as a gentle hint and which may be sufficient. It saves the apparently offended from loss of face he would incur if he made an explicit accusation which turned out to be unjustified. The 'priming' move may be achieved entirely non-verbally: assertive stance (high tonus, high head position, eye contact, frowning); moving forward, jostling, possibly touching. Or it could include a verbal request which obliquely refers to the apparent wrong, e.g. a rhetorical question with an obvious literal meaning ('Excuse me, are you in a hurry?), but the implied meaning 'Why are you queue jumping?'

Response:

> A successful assertion move would be followed by a reversal of action, an apology and an excuse such as, 'I am sorry, I did not realise you were queueing.' This can be followed by the remainder of the apology sequence, namely relief and mini-misation. An apology or excuse without a reversal of action would be followed by a different second move, as follows:

Second move:

> *Elements:* Vocal and non-verbal – as for assertive attitude. Verbal: 'I think I was before you' plus 'I'm in a hurry, too'. *Function:* To make clear the transgression and to make clear the excuse was not acceptable. The offended person is by this stage no longer in an ambiguous situation and can assert 'the rules of the game', namely that he has the right to X, that

the other has taken it from him, that he insists on his right and is not prepared to give it up. The second move can be used in any situation where there is a clear transgression of rights, e.g. where a service has been requested but not fulfilled ('I ordered a rare steak, not an overdone one; please could you change it.' 'I didn't ask for an engine overhaul – just a tune up; I don't see why I should pay for what I didn't ask for.' 'This X you sold me is faulty; please can I have my money back.'). The move can also be used to turn down an unreasonable request ('I'm sorry but I was here first and I'm in a hurry too.'). Note that this move is more assertive – more clearly a demand – than the first, but still leaves open the possibility of a justification.

Response:

A further apology or elaborated excuse, with reversal of action, or a challenge that any rights have been transgressed. These are all 'legal' moves in the game. A remedy without restoration of substance and insufficient justification or a groundless challenge lead to the third assertion move. (Conversely, a substantive remedy, a sufficient justification or a legitimate challenge will lead to giving relief or an apology on the part of the asserter.)

Third move:

This is an explicit demand to the offender to restore the situation (return or replace goods or money, reverse an act). A threat of retribution is made: 'Kindly do X or else . . . I shall do it/complain to the Y/take legal action', etc). Ultimately the force of the demand is dependent on the threat of the retribution being realistic.

The therapist then summarises: 'There is an important rule to remember in asserting our rights. Usually this kind of assertion involves communicating something negative, e.g. 'stop behaving that way'. This should be done at first in an implicit way – hint at it, use non-verbal cues, and if this fails make it more and more explicit – put it into words, make demands, ask for an apology, and remain pleasant, reasonable and persuasive. This puts the other in the role of behaving likewise.

REFUSAL (Exercise 45)

Patients are now asked to imagine situations where they think they would like to refuse requests. They should then ask whether they think the request is unreasonable. Could the other justify making the request on the grounds of friendship or the situation?

A situation is taken in which the question of the 'reasonableness' of the request is an open one, but the individual wishes to turn it down.

First move:

> As before, the refusal should be a cautious one, since the request may not be unreasonable, e.g. in asking for a date, giving an explicit excuse. Use of non-verbal cues is important, e.g. withholding of 'immediacy' cues.

Second move:

> This may be a repeat of the first move, depending on the situation.

Third move:

> If unsuccessful, the refusal is made more explicit by the withholding of a justifying account ('I'm sorry, no') with the use of assertion cues.

Fourth move:

> If unsuccessful, the refusal is made more explicit ('I don't want to'), and the transgression pointed out ('I've said no – you're pushing your luck too far'). A possible threat may be necessary.

The escalation to explicit refusal and rejection is justified because the requester breaks the rule of respect for personal rights and is therefore no longer 'reasonable'.

Therapists demonstrate Exercise 45. This is followed with examples of suitable situations for further modelling and role-play and should be obtained from the patients – events which have recently happened or could happen to them. After the patients have completed a few sequences satisfactorily, participants should work through them again rapidly, to speed up response reflexes. During these faster routines, special attention should be paid to the sticking points, where the patient may respond with a reflex from his customary behaviour pattern.

References

ALBERTI, R. E. AND EMMONS, M. L. (1973) *Your Perfect Right*. California: Impact.

GOFFMAN, E. (1972) *Relations in Public : Micro-studies of the Public Order*. Harmondsworth: Penguin.

HARRÉ, R. AND SECORD, C. W. (1972) *The Explanation of Social Behaviour*. Oxford: Blackwell.

KENDON, A. AND FERBER, A. (1973) A description of some human greetings. In R. P. Michael and J. H. Cook (eds) *Comparative Ecology and Behaviour of Primates*. London: Academic Press.

ROBINSON, P. (1972) *Language and Social Behaviour*. Harmondsworth: Penguin.

9. Tactics and strategies

Briefing

This section deals with the cognitive – or problem solving – stage, the selection and putting together of responses in sequences which will be effective in obtaining desired social goals. 'Tactics' are used in the smallscale minute-by-minute action decisions made on the basis of continuous feedback from the other, and 'strategies' are used for higher-order and longer-term plans which may span several encounters.

Tactics

Presentation

'Everyone has now developed a wider repertoire of social skills, which means that they should be able to choose alternative ways, better ways, new ways of responding to others during the minute-by-minute flow of conversation. Unfortunately, this is not easy. Firstly, we have all got life-long habits of responding-without-thinking, and secondly, everything happens at split-second speed in conversation, and there is little time to stop and think. So one problem is: We know what to do, but by the time we remember to do it, it's too late. In this session we shall look at ways of breaking down old bad habits, and of putting choice back into our behaviour.

'First, in any conversation or interaction there are *choice points* –

the time between the other stopping and before you start speaking. Second, at those choice points, there are a number of *alternative* ways to respond, and these should be considered. Third, one of these alternatives is *chosen*, and this should be one that is effective.

'There are three pitfalls: Failing to consider alternatives, failing to choose (by responding out of habit), and failing to select one of the better responses.'

Training may be organised as follows: A situation is described (supplied or obtained from patients). A patient is asked to give a number of alternative responses to the situation and evaluate each of these. The patient is then asked to consider the alternatives suggested by the therapists or patients and evaluate each of them. Finally, one is selected as the most effective (with guidance) and the sequence role-played and rehearsed in the usual way. Therapists demonstrate with the first example below, and patients then work through further examples, as suggested in Exercise 47.

CHOOSING A RESPONSE (from Goldsmith and McFall 1975)

Let's suppose you respond to an employment ad in the newspaper and go for an interview. A tall, well-dressed man walks up to you in the waiting room. He thinks you are someone else and says, 'You must be Mr X, the new man from down the hall.'

Alternatives	Evaluations
'Yes, I am'	Wrong
'I am looking for so and so'	Neutral
'I am Mr Y. I would like to apply for the job'	Neutral
'I don't know who Mr X is, but I am not he. I am looking for a job interview'	Neutral
'No, I'm not. I am here in response to the ad for employment'	Neutral
'No, I am sorry, I am not the man. I am so and so. I am here for an interview'	Right

After a few examples have been worked through the process of giving alternatives and choosing is speeded up.

Another version of this technique for ordinary conversation is to get two patients to talk and to stop the interaction at various points. The last speaker is then asked to suggest alternative responses, to evaluate them, choose one and continue with the response chosen. The therapists demonstrate and patients work through Exercise 48.

Strategies

REWARDING, CONTROLLING AND PRESENTING SELF

This section brings together those skills from earlier parts of the manual which have a common purpose or goal, such as rewarding or controlling the other, or creating good impressions. It therefore serves as a revision exercise.

Presentation

'In addition to the decisions we make at each choice-point, we have to decide on an approach or strategy over a whole conversation or series of conversations. We have to plan ahead with a goal and the situation in mind, and we put together a strategy using the repertoire of skills at our disposal. We will discuss, first, a strategy for *rewarding* the other – to get him interested, talking and responding more, to feel more friendly towards you; next, one for *controlling* the other – to get him to talk less or about different things and reduce his control of you and the situation; finally, a strategy for *presenting oneself* to the other effectively.'

REWARDING OTHERS (Exercise 49)

The therapists demonstrate the following steps in a relevant, role-played situation such as consolidating a friendship or rewarding someone for a positive achievement or a kindly gesture. Obviously the order of the steps should be varied somewhat to suit the situation chosen.

Step 1.   Select a 'target' other and get some information about him and his interests. Evaluate the situation and decide on your goal.

Step 2.   On sighting, greet the other.

Step 3.   Use the GSF (general-specific-feeling) question routine, with not-too-personal questions (e.g. about health, recent activities).

Step 4.   Use the full range of listener responses.

Step 5.   Make fairly personal self-disclosures of reasonable length, and personalise your style of language.

· Step 6.   Disclose feelings, opinions and beliefs of similarity, and use non-verbal expressiveness.

Step 7.   Colour and emphasise your talk with non-verbal accompaniments.

Step 8.   Use immediacy cues, particularly gaze and positive expressions and good vocal tone.

Step 9.   Mesh smoothly, avoiding interruptions and non-response. Use mainly implicit (non-verbal) hand-over and taking-up cues and don't resist turn offers or suppress turn claims.

Step 10. Use supportive routines, especially compliments, praise and sympathy and thanks. Make offers and invitations.

Therapists model the full sequence, not necessarily using everything, but only as the drift of the conversation allows. Patients try this in work triads, the monitor ticking off points as they are covered. The same procedure is followed for the steps below.

CONTROLLING OTHERS (Exercise 50)
The therapist should again provide a demonstration, such as controlling an over-dominant person in a social or work situation.

Step 1.   Get information about the other, and situation, and decide on your goal.

Step 2.   On sighting, greet the other.

Step 3.   Use the GSF question routine plus some more searching questions.

Step 4.   Use fewer reflections and attention signals but more non-verbal listener comments such as questioning and surprise expressions.

Step 5.   Speak at length but make self-disclosures less personal *or* speak briefly and factually.

Step 6.   Make disclosures of 'difference' and change topic of conversation.

Step 7.   Disclose opinions and beliefs more than feelings, and make less use of non-verbal emotion expressions.

Step 8.   Use non-verbal emphasis and colour more.

Step 9.   Use dominance cues, particularly more gaze early in the conversation, and break gaze last; use critical expression (frowning brow), loud and resonant voice, *or* use coldness cues, such as gaze aversion, orienting away.

Step 10.   Use interruptions and non-response. Keep the initiative in verbal exchanges by handing over and taking up the conversation, and by suppressing turn offers and resisting turn claims.

Step 11.   Make requests, give advice, make refusals and assert right, but resist apologies – all where appropriate only.

Step 12.   In extreme case, use negative attitude cues.

A final exercise combines the two forms, with rewarding responses being interspersed with controlling ones, such as

1.   Full listener responses, good meshing and 'immediacy' cues, followed by

2.   Interrupting, disclosure of difference and 'dominance' cues etc.

PRESENTING SELF (Exercise 51)

'We can partly control the impression others have of us by managing our physical appearance and our behaviour. There are many impressions we should try to convey, but three in particular: attractiveness, status and likeability. For attractiveness, we can manage our physical appearance and non-verbal behaviour; for status, we can, in addition disclose our positive achievements, and use more controlling skills; and for likeability we can use rewarding skills.'

A demonstration role-play for this exercise might be going out on a date, going for a job interview or meeting someone important. Again, the order would be changed to suit the situation.

Step 1. Prepare physical appearance, particularly clothes, hair and make-up (as appropriate) to enhance physical attractiveness and status.

Step 2. While initiating encounter, maintain gaze, erect body tonus, direct orientation, voice volume and clarity.

Step 3. Mask non-verbal expressions of emotional states like anxiety, depression and feelings of inferiority, with socially sanctioned expressions like the social smile and the elements in Step 2.

Step 4. Make indirect disclosures of status enhancing facts about self (interesting job, girl/boyfriend, spouse, family, spare-time interests, achievements) and with-hold negative information (loneliness, failures, emotional problems etc.).

Step 5. Be rewarding where possible.

Step 6. Be controlling where appropriate.

It is sometimes useful to get patients to make a list of all their positive attributes (Step 4) and to role-play talking about these before the whole routine is tried.

Revision

The next exercise (Exercise 52) is a revision exercise designed to combine both strategies and tactics, the principle being that the responses selected at the various choice points in the interaction are based on the other's last comment and one's own longer-term strategy. At this point, we pick up the theme of the attitude expression section and put it into the wider context of strategies and tactics, as follows:

First, what is the other's attitude to me? e.g. superior

Second, what strategy is he using? e.g. controlling

Third, what strategy shall I use? counter-control

Fourth, what control tactic shall I use at this point?

To illustrate, we give an example dialogue from an actual training session, with a blow-by-blow account of the tactics involved.

This can be role-played between therapists for demonstration purposes.

Pete and Derek are 'comps' in a printing works. It is about mid-morning, and Pete comes over to Derek for a quick break and chat. Pete is an extravert and quite dominant, Derek rather a submissive person. Pete says loudly and boisterously:

(P's 1st move):	'Hello there, Derek.'
D:	'Oh, hello.'
P's 2nd move:	'How are you goin' then?'
D:	'All right, thanks.'
P's 3rd move:	'Strugglin' then, are you?'
D:	'Yeah. I'm always strugglin'; it's always a struggle.'
P's 4th move:	'Getting you down then, is it?'
D:	'Yeah' (despondently). 'Can't seem to get to grips with it.'
P's 5th move:	'Rotten job then, is it?'
D:	'Yeah, always gets the rotten jobs.'
P's 6th move:	(interrupting) 'You don't want to let them push you around, mate.'

Pete's moves can be analysed as a dominance sequence as follows:

P's 1st move:	Starts control strategy by initiating greeting, which makes a response obligatory.
D's response:	Compliance.
P's 2nd move:	Consolidate greeting. Continues by making formal disclosure obligatory.
D's response:	Compliance.
P's 3rd move:	Continues with (i) question (making answer obligatory) and (ii) implication of weakness in other.
D's response:	Compliance to (i), double acceptance of (ii).
P's 4th move:	Repeats.
D's response:	Repetition of compliance to 3rd move.

P's 5th move: Repeats.

D's response: Repetition of compliance to 4th move.

P's 6th move: Continues with (i) interruption and (ii) giving advice.

The task of training is to get Derek to break the control sequence, to *choose* his responses, instead of responding out of habit. The following tactics are an example of an overall strategy which might be termed a counter-control sequence.

P's 1st move: 'Hello there, Derek.'

D: 'Hello Peter, *how are you?*'

P's 2nd move: 'Fine, mate, fine. You strugglin' then?'

D: *'No more'n usual, Pete. How about you?'*

P's 3rd move: 'Yeah, OK yeah. What's this, then? Rotten job they've give you 'ere, ain't it?'

D: *'Better than havin' nothin' to do, in't it?'*

Analysis

P's 1st move: Starts control strategy by initiating greeting, which makes a response obligatory.

D's response: Obliges, *but counters by making a formal disclosure* obligatory.

P's 2nd move: Obliges but tries new tactic with (i) question (making answer obligatory) and (ii) implication of weakness in other.

D's response: Obliges but *counters with (i) minimisation of implication of weakness and (ii) further question.*

P's 3rd move: Minimal obligatory answer but tries again with (i) question and (ii) another implication.

D's response: *Obligatory answer but counters with (i) question which is also (ii) counter-implication.*

In summary, then, D counters P's control tactics by getting back part of the *initiative* (the second move of the greeting sequence), by asking *questions* and by *counter-implications*. Other tactics can be used, such as denials, demands for accounts, etc.

After role-playing the above interaction, the patient should then present his own scene and attempt to generate his own counter-control moves. In this way he learns he has a *choice* of strategies, and does not have to comply with one which the other tries to impose.

References

SPIVACK, G. AND SHURE, M. B. (1974) *Social Adjustment of Young Children: A cognitive Approach to solving Real Life Problems.* San Francisco, Cal., Washington and London: Jossey-Bass.

GOLDSMITH, J. B. AND MCFALL, R. M. (1975). Development and evaluation of an interpersonal training program for psychiatric inpatients. *Journal Abnormal Psychology*, 84, 51–8.

10.   Situation training

As mentioned in the introduction, our attention should now turn to problems experienced in specific situations. Our usual procedure is as follows:

Each patient in turn is asked to describe in detail a specific problem situation, a description of which he should have written down previously in his diary. He 'casts' other patients and the therapists in the roles of the people involved in the situation, and arranges the furniture and other props. With the aid of the diary description, he gives the participants thumbnail sketches of these other individuals – their age, social class, status, personality and behavioural characteristics – and gives an outline of the dialogue. The patient 'plays' himself, but at various points may role-reverse with other participants to give them a better idea of their character. The first simulation is acted out as closely as possible to the original event, and this should be videotaped. The videotape is played back, and the patient notes, and others suggest, alternative strategies, or a number of points for correction. If necessary, another participant can role-reverse with the patient, to give him a more objective view of his own performance. Other participants now try out their suggested strategies, and the patient evaluates each of these and chooses one for further practice. After a satisfactory performance has been achieved, the group, or part of the group, can move to a more realistic setting, such as a canteen, restaurant or pub, and the exercise can be repeated.

A wide variety of situations can be simulated and practised in this way, and many of our own patients report that they are able to remember and replicate the rehearsed performance in their own environments quite successfully. Examples include: A clerk of the court addressing magistrates, a managing director meeting hostile members of another board of directors, an accountant excusing himself to be sick at a formal dinner, a young man talking to a girl in a pub and inviting her to play bar billiards, a photographer presenting his portfolio at an interview, a student talking to other students in a brightly lit lecture theatre, and so on. [This concludes the therapist's manual. We give below a suggested handbook for patients.]

11.   Trainee's handbook

Introducing social skills training

We now know from research evidence that a lot of the problems people have are due to, or are aggravated by, a lack of social skills. Some people get depressed and lonely because they lack the skills to make friends and hold conversations. Some panic and withdraw because they lack skills for coping with people who make them nervous. Some feel inferior and helpless because they can't assert themselves or deal with people who try to dominate them. Social skills training aims to help people use their skills better or learn new ones, and we consider it a form of education rather than 'treatment'.

Training is carried out by instructors who teach what the skills are; by 'rehearsal' of these skills at weekly training sessions; and by trying it out in real life in the form of homework assignments. The topics covered include improving one's powers of observation and accurate judgment; basic conversation skills such as listening, asking questions and talking; expressiveness skills such as the use of body language in showing how one feels; social techniques for special situations, such as starting conversations with strangers, asserting one's rights, and so on.

We ask trainees to make a commitment by agreeing to attend sessions regularly and to carry out the 'homework'. We also give our assurance that no tasks will be impossibly difficult or frightening, though they will get progressively harder. Finally, and to emphasise the point, we urge trainees to think of training as a form of education rather than treatment, and to carry out the exercises and assignments as they would when learning any other new skill.

Description of this guide

This guide consists of exercises, homework assignments and information about effective social skills. The *exercises* consist of a number of steps, or guidepoints, for a particular task, like a brief conversation. The exercises will be used during the training sessions. The *homework assignments* are divided into two parts: *Preparation* and *task*. The preparation usually involves writing out lists of information and instructions on pocket-sized filing cards, which should be carried around and referred to before and after carrying out a task, or better still, learned off by heart. The task is what you actually do. We would like you to carry out the tasks as often as you can, and at least once a day (unless otherwise stated). We would also like you to note the results in a daily diary, and to summarise the results for the week on a homework form.

Materials

You will need a pocket-sized Dataday type diary. You should 'write it up' at the end of the day or last thing at night. The kind of information you should put in your diary should be as follows:

(a) Anything that happened to you that was interesting, amusing, annoying and so on.
(b) Anything that made you feel very nervous or depressed.
(c) The results of carrying out your assignments, as described above.

You will also need a wad of medium sized file cards. Instructions how to use these will be given in each of the homework assignments and by the instructor.

Basic conversation

BRIEF CONVERSATION

Many of the difficulties people have are concerned with starting conversations, and keeping them going. The introductory exercise is a complete but very brief conversation.

Exercise 1
1. Turn to the person next to you.
2. Greet him.
3. Ask a couple of questions.
4. Answer any questions.
5. Close conversation.

LONGER CONVERSATION

We can add to or change this basic format to deal with special difficulties. The second exercise includes 3 extra points.

Exercise 2
1. Turn to the other person next to you.
2. Identify his attitude (i.e. does he seem to want to talk?).
3. If negative, greet him and stop.
4. If positive, greet him and continue.
5. Ask three questions, the last one specific.
6. Give listener responses.
7. Answer any questions.
8. Volunteer information about self (e.g. work, home).
9. Close conversation.

SUMMARY

We can add to and change the basic format in many ways, and many of these ways will be described in the coming training sessions. We now ask you to make up a conversation for your homework assignment.

HOMEWORK ASSIGNMENT 1

Preparation
Fill in the missing steps in the task (below). For instance, for step 5 you could write 'Make comment about weather' and for step 6 'Ask a question . . .' Then write out the list of steps on a file card, and label this Task Card 1, CONVERSATION. Carry this around, refer to it before and after carrying out the task. Also, be sure to describe some difficult situations in your diaries. We shall need this information next session.

The task
1. Sight someone you recognise (e.g. in the street, at work).
2. Identify his attitude.
3. If negative, greet him and stop.
4. If positive, greet him and continue.
5.
6.
7.
8.
9. Take your leave.

Observation

PROBLEM SITUATIONS

To develop effective social skills, we need to be good observers of situations and other people. Poor observation leads to mis-understanding, doing the wrong thing, upsetting people or being upset ourselves and not knowing what to do in situations. We start by looking at situations that have gone wrong, to see how poor observation might have contributed to the problem.

Exercise 3
1. Describe a recent social problem, e.g. talking to strangers.
2. Give an example, e.g. a recent party (refer to your diary).

INFORMATION

We need two kinds of information about such a problem situation: Facts on the one hand, feelings and attitudes on the other. Exercise 4 is about the facts.

Exercise 4
1. Describe situation:
   time of day,
   place – town, street,
   type of situation – shopping, coffee break, interview,
   physical features and conditions – description of room, shop, etc., and conditions – whether crowded, stuffy, bright etc.
2. Describe people present:
   number present,

names, ages, sex, personality, physical appearance, role
(mother, boss, workmate), interests,
anything else you may know about them.

3. What happened, or did not happen:
events,
actions,
conversations.

4. What were you feeling?

FEELINGS AND ATTITUDES
As well as the facts we need to know what people feel and believe,
and we find this out by observing what they do – the social signals –
and by checking our impressions with those of others.

Exercise 5
1. Identify one individual in the situation (name).
2. What attitude or feeling was he expressing –
    (a) in general
    (b) to you (look at attitudes listed below)?
3. How did you get these impressions (go through the social
    signals listed below)?
4. Did others agree with you? Ask them.
5. What alternative impressions might you have formed?
6. How sure are you now about your first impression?

List of some attitudes, styles and feelings
These are some of the ways we describe each other's attitudes,
styles and feelings. You can use as many or few as you like to
describe someone.
Warm or cold
Dominant or submissive
Socially anxious or relaxed
Happy or sad
Rewarding or unrewarding
Controlling or uncontrolling
Feminine or masculine
Attractive or unattractive
Passive or active
Difficult or easy
Emotional or unemotional
Socially skilled or unskilled

List of social signals

These are some of the signals we observe – often unconsciously – when forming impressions of another person's feelings, attitudes, personality and so on. We will return to them in more detail later.

Physical appearance	Size
	Height
	Hair (length, colour)
	Face (features, complexion)
	Dress
	Cosmetics, etc.
Vocal	Loud or soft
	Resonant or thin tone
	High, low or varied pitch
	Distinct or slurred
	Fast or slow pace
	Many or few speech errors such as stammering.
Conversation	Lengthy or brief
	General or detailed
	Personal or impersonal
	Varied or monotonous
	Humorous or lacking in humour
	Colourful or dull
	Good or poor listener
	Smooth or rough
	Assertive or compliant
	Supportive or unsupportive.
Non-Verbal	Positive, negative or blank facial expression
	Frequent or rare looking
	Physically close or distant
	Turned towards or away
	Posture upright or slumped
	closed or open
	forward or backward
	tense or relaxed
	Frequent or few gestures.

CAUSES

Exercise 5 is a 'check-out' routine, that is, a way of checking out the accuracy of our judgments. We need to do this to avoid making the wrong judgment about people. But it is also important to know why people express certain attitudes and beliefs. If someone looks cross, is it because of me, or the situation, his personality, his mood, or what? If we don't ask why, we may take it personally, and that may be a serious mistake.

Exercise 6
1. Identify someone's attitude or feeling.
2. *Why* is he feeling that way? Because of –
   The situation?
   His personality?
   His mood?
   Someone else?
   Me?
3. Ask others.

SELF-OBSERVATION

We have looked at how we may form wrong impressions about others. Now we deal with how others form wrong impressions about us, and how we might be sending out the wrong social signals.

Exercise 7
1. What feeling or attitude did you want to express
   (a) in general?
   (b) to the other?
2. Did you succeed in putting this across? What impression did you make?
3. Check out your social signals.
4. Do others agree with you?
5. Do you still think you succeeded, and if not, why not?
6. List the social signals you would like to change.

SUMMARY

We have seen how we come to misunderstand each other, by misinterpreting other's signals or sending the wrong ones ourselves. We need to practise these exercises in real life to improve our observation skills.

Preparation
Write out the list of attitudes on a file card, and do the same for the list of social signals. Call this Cue Card 1, SOCIAL SIGNALS. Write out the steps for the task (below) on a third card, and entitle this Cue Card 2, OBSERVATION.

The task
1. Carry out the conversation task – Card 1.
2. Watch the situation carefully.
3. Note the other's attitude to you.
4. Watch his behaviour (social signals) carefully and check and correct your first impression.
5. Check your own attitude and behaviour carefully (social signals).

FACE CUES OF EMOTION

We have looked at social signals – yours and the other person's – in a general way. Now we shall look at them rather more closely. This will help in both observing and using social signals more skilfully. First we'll look at the expression of emotion. The next exercise deals with how to read people's faces better.

Exercise 8

Partner A	*Partner* B
1. Select 2 or 3 facial cues of one emotion and express these	Guess the emotion expressed and the cues your partner is using
2. Select 1 facial cue and express this	Guess the emotion and cue used
3. Select 1 cue from 2 different emotions and express this as a 'blend'	Guess the emotions and cues used

List of face cues

To recognise or express this feeling:	You can use these face cues:		
	Brow region	*Eye region*	*Mouth region*
Surprise/ Interest	brows raised	eyes wide open	mouth open, relaxed
Fear	brows drawn together and raised	eyes wide	mouth corners drawn back
Anger	brows lowered, 'knotted'	eyes wide	lips pressed or 'squared'
Disgust/ Contempt	brows lowered	nose 'screwed up'	upper lips curled
Sadness	brows lowered at corners	eyes lowered	mouth corners down
Happiness	neutral	'bagging' under eyes, 'crows feet' creases	mouth corners up

VOICE CUES OF EMOTION

The next exercise deals with detecting emotion in the voice.

Exercise 9

Partner A	*Partner* B
1. Select 2 or 3 vocal cues of an emotion and express these	Guess the emotion and cues used
2. Select 1 vocal cue only and express this	Guess the emotion and cue used
3. Select a cue from 2 different emotions and express these as a vocal 'blend'	Guess the emotions and cues used

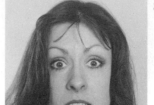

Surprise

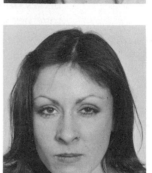

Anger

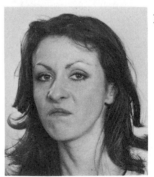

Disgust

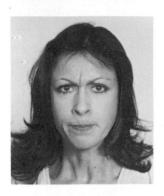

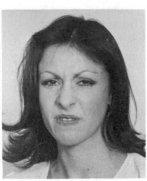

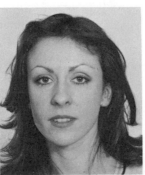

Neutral

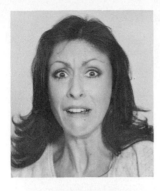 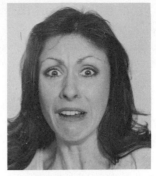 Fear

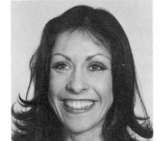 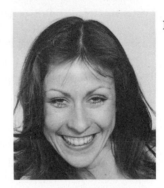 Happiness

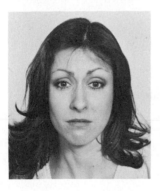 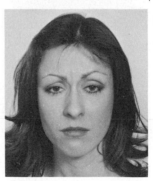 Sadness

Expressions of emotion in the face

The face is the most important region for expressing and detecting emotion. We give here two examples each of the six primary expressions and one neutral. Identify the facial cues used in each one from the list given on page 269. Use the neutral expression for comparison.

4. Select a face cue and a   Guess the emotions and cues
    voice cue and express these   used
    together

List of voice cues

To recognise or
express this feeling: You can use these voice cues:

Surprise/Interest   high, varied pitch
                       fast
                       rising inflection (as in question)

Fear   varied volume
                       varied pitch
                       rising inflection

Anger   loud
                       high
                       harsh
                       clipped
                       rising and falling inflection

Disgust   slow
                       slurred

Sadness   soft
                       low
                       slow
                       falling inflection
                       slurred

Happiness   fairly loud
                       fairly high, variable
                       fast
                       rising inflection

ATTITUDE CUES

We can also tell what the other person's attitude is – whether he
likes us and so on, from special signals he uses and which we can
learn to detect.

Exercise 10

Partner A	Partner B
1. Choose an attitude (warm, cold, assertive or submissive) and express this to your partner using as many cues as you can	Guess the cues your partner is using
2. Select one or two cues only and express these	Guess the cues your partner is using
3. Select two or three cues from two *different* attitudes and express these	Guess the two attitudes your partner is expressing and the cues used.

List of attitude cues (seated positions)

Warm, friendly

Face :	Positive expressions – e.g. interest, smiling
Gaze :	Long and frequent looks and eye contact
Voice :	Soft, low, resonant
Distance :	Fairly close (within three feet)
Touch :	Hand on arm
Position :	About 45 degree angle to other person
Orientation :	Head and shoulders towards each other
Posture :	Open arms and partially open or loosely crossed legs
	Forward lean or moderate sideways lean
	General movement
Speech :	Listener responses
	Speaker disclosures of similarity
	Few speech disturbances
	Good timing
	Handing over conversation

It is helpful as an aid to remembering the non-verbal cues for warm/friendly to think of them as 'immediacy' cues, bringing you psychologically closer to the other – more looking, physical closeness and direct orientation, open posture, etc. Cold/unfriendly attitudes are communicated by the reverse – more distance between the partners, as well as less conversation, meshing and so on.

Assertive/dominant

Face : Relaxed, neutral face or frowning
Gaze : Fewer, but longer, looks. Breaks gaze last
Voice : Loud, deep tone
Distance : Either fairly close or fairly distant
Orientation : Either face to face or turned more than 45 degrees away
Posture : Reclining angle, relaxed, limbs sprawled, shoulders squared, chest expanded, head raised (high tonus)
Speech : Few reflections
Speaks at length
Quick responses and interruptions
Asks questions and changes topic
Initiates and closes interaction
Expresses different opinions

Combined

Face : Mixed sequence, smiling and frowning
Gaze : Looks long and often
Voice : Moderately loud, resonant, low
Distance : Fairly close
Position : About 45 degree angle to other person
Posture : Open style
Forward or sideways lean
Relaxed
High tonus
Speech Full listener responses
Speaks at length
Few speech disturbances
Expresses both similar and different opinions
Good timing, quick responses
Handing over

Negative or anxious (for information only)

A look and turning away
Looking 'through'
Turning away from someone about to talk
Defensive posture or standing too close
Recoiling or flinching

Frowning with head forward or up or back
Self-grooming or picking clothes and frowning
Sudden glance and alerted posture
Vulgar gestures, finger shaking

SUMMARY

People communicate their feelings and attitudes by special
signals or cues – of the face, voice and body. We can improve our
ability to detect and express feelings and attitudes by learning
and practising these cues. At this stage we are simply learning
what they are – later we shall practise them.

HOMEWORK ASSIGNMENT 3

Preparation
Write out a 'Cue Card 2, EMOTIONS' listing the face and voice cues
for showing feelings, and a 'Cue Card 3, ATTITUDES', listing the
verbal and non-verbal cues for expressing attitudes. Write on
another card the steps of the task (below) and call this Task Card
3, OBSERVATION.

The task
1. Carry out the conversation and observation tasks on Cards
   1 and 2.
2. Watch the other person carefully and look for the face cues for
   showing feelings.
3. Listen for the voice cues for showing feelings.
4. Watch for the verbal and non-verbal cues for expressing
   attitudes.

Listening

We need good observation skills in conversation. We need to
know what the other is feeling to be a good listener, and we need
to be a good listener so that the other will want to talk to us. This
section is about just that – good listening skills.

REFLECTING

The first listener skill builds on the last session – understanding
the messages the other person is sending you, then letting him
know you understand. This listener skill is called reflecting, or
'saying back', i.e. saying back what the other said in your own

words. This tells the speaker that you understand, and makes him feel you are interested.

Exercise 11
1. Choose a partner and ask him to talk about something.
2. Listen carefully to what he says.
3. Identify the feeling, belief or opinion expressed (if any).
4. Identify the facts being described.
5. Say it back, using this special sentence, 'You feel (think, believe) . . . because (reason)'.

REFLECTING NON-VERBAL EXPRESSIONS
We can reflect or say back more accurately if we attend to the important cues of face and voice.

Exercise 12
1. As before, listen to your partner and identify the feeling etc. expressed.
2. Listen and look for the face and voice cues.
3. Identify the facts being described.
4. Say it back as before.

Cues to listen and look for

Face		Voice	
Eyebrows:	High or low position? Shape?	*Volume:*	Loud, soft or varied?
Forehead:	Lined or wrinkled?	*Pitch:*	High, low or varied?
Eyes:	Wide open or narrowed? Direction of gaze?	*Tone:*	Blaring, resonant, thin?
Eyelids:	Tense or relaxed?	*Pace:*	Fast or slow?
Mouth:	Open or closed?	*Inflection:*	Upward or downward? Regular or irregular?
Lips:	Curved up or down? Pulled back or pushed forward?	*Rhythm:*	Regular or irregular?
	Tense or relaxed?	*Clarity:*	Clipped or slurred?

MOODMATCHING
A good listener is responsive to the other person – if he smiles, the listener smiles; if he looks serious, the listener looks serious.

This is called moodmatching. We practise this by 'doing what the speaker does'.

Exercise 13
As Exercise 12, plus
5. Match the speaker's non-verbal expression (face and voice).

REFLECTING ACCURATELY

A good listener is also good at finding just the right word to sum up what the other feels. The technique is to identify the general feeling, then try to identify the particular feeling.

Exercise 14
1. As before, listen to your partner and identify the *general* feeling expressed.
2. Identify the *particular* feeling expressed.
3. Identify the facts being described.
4. Reflect back the *particular* feelings (use special sentence for reflecting).

List of general and particular emotion words

General:	*Angry*	*Happy*	*Sad*	*Fear*
Particular:	Annoyed	Pleased	Disappointed	Anxious
	Enraged	Satisfied	Sorry	Alarmed
	Irritated	Relieved	Hurt	Worried
		Delighted	Regretful	Uncertain
				Confused

General:	*Disgust*	*Surprise/Interest*
	Contemptuous	Amazed
Particular:	Sickened	Curious
	Shocked	Intrigued
	Revolted	Fascinated

OTHER LISTENER RESPONSES

We don't reflect back all the time when listening – we just nod, say 'mhmm', 'yeah', 'I see' and so on. This is what we call attention feedback, because you are giving your attention and interest. This is rewarding to the speaker – he will talk more. The less attention feedback, the less he will talk.

Exercise 15
As Exercise 14, except
4. wait for the speaker to pause and look up.
5. respond using one of the following:

Small responses	Nod head
	'Mhmm'
	'Yes/Yeah'.
Medium responses	'I see'
	'I know what you mean'
Full response (reflections)	'You feel . . . because . . .'

SUMMARY

We have looked at some of the things a good listener does to 'reward' the speaker, show him you understand and care, and how to be a more sensitive listener. We need to practise these things every time someone talks to us.

HOMEWORK ASSIGNMENT 4

Preparation
Write out a 'Cue Card 4, EMOTION WORDS', listing the general and particular emotion words. Also write out the task (below) on a card and entitle this 'Task Card 4, LISTENING'.

The task
1. Carry out the conversation and observation tasks (Cards 1, 2, 3).
2. While the other person talks, use some or all of the following listener responses:

Small responses	Head nod, 'Mhmm', 'Yes/Yeah'
Medium responses	'I see', 'I know what you mean'
Full responses	'You feel/felt . . . because . . .'
	Or reflect in your own words
Non-verbal responses	Mirror other's expression.

LISTENER COMMENT

As listeners we don't just reflect and attend to what the other is saying. We also comment or disclose our own feelings and beliefs, which may be the same as, or different from, the speaker's.

Exercise 16
1. Choose a partner and get him to talk to you about something.
2. Listen carefully to what he says (facts and feelings).
3. Disclose feeling of similarity ('I also feel . . . because . . .')
4. Disclose feeling of difference ('But I feel . . . because . . .')

MORE LISTENER COMMENT

We sometimes agree, sometimes disagree, with the speaker. We sometimes feel pleased, sometimes annoyed, sometimes interested, sometimes bored with what he is saying. We can *show* these things by face and voice, or *tell* him in words.

Exercise 17
1. While listening to the other person, show you agree, then disagree.
2. Show you are pleased, then displeased.
3. Show you are interested, then bored.
4. Show you are puzzled, then surprised.

QUESTIONING

The listener skills above will encourage the other to talk more, but won't get him started. For this we need questions. We usually start with *general* questions, go on to *specific* ones and finally on to *feeling* questions, that is questions that ask what the other thinks, believes, feels about something. We can also ask *open* rather than *closed* questions.

Exercise 18
1. Turn to the list *Questions – topics and examples.*
2. Ask a general question (a), topic (1)
3, Ask a specific question (b), topic (1)
4. Ask a feeling question (c), topic (1)
5. Repeat with another aspect of topic (1) or
6. Repeat this time with topic (2)

Questions – topics and examples

Topics	Example questions
1. Anything the other person has been involved in recently.	(a) General: 'What are you doing at the moment?' 'What's been happening recently?' 'How are things going?'

	(b) Specific	'What did you do exactly?'
	(c) Feeling	'What was that like?'
		'Were you angry/surprised?'

2. Things he is doing, has done, or belongs to
   (i) work
   (ii) home
   (iii) travel
   (iv) hobbies
   (v) social

(a) General:	'How's work going?'
	'How are things at home?'
(b) Specific:	'What do you do exactly?'
	'How's your baby?'
(c) Feeling:	'What's it like?'
	'Do you find it interesting?'
	'Do you get . . . (annoyed/fed up)?

3. Things in common
   (i) being 'here'
   (ii) TV, cinema, pubs
   (iii) cars, hi-fi
   (iv) people (friends and acquaintances)

(a) General:	'Have you been here before?'
	'Have you seen any good films recently?'
(b) specific:	'What did you do here last time?'
	'What was . . . (film) . . . about?'
(c) Feeling:	'Did you like . . . (being here, new car)?' 'What do you think of . . . (this place etc.)?'

4. Current local and national topics
   (i) news, gossip
   (ii) sport
   (iii) personalities
   (iv) forthcoming events

(a) General:	'Anything happening this week?'
(b) Specific:	'Are you going to . . . (event)?'
(c) Feeling:	'What do you think it will be like?'

REVISION

In the revision exercise below we bring all the above points together in the form of a complete conversation, rather like we did in the introductory session. There are two things we do in this (and all) conversations – make *decisions* and carry out *actions*. We go through the exercise step by step.

Exercise 19
This is what you decide

This is what you can do
(some examples)

1. Pick someone you could talk to   ———
2. Decide what his attitude is (e.g. friendly)   Observe his non-verbal behaviour

3. Decide what your attitude   Prepare and watch your own
   is going to be (e.g. friendly)   behaviour (Don't forget to:
                                   a. check that what you do is
                                      relevant to the situation.
                                   b. check you are giving out
                                      the right message).

4. Choose a style of greeting   Greet him
5. Choose one kind of question   Ask him general, factual
                                   question
6. Listen to what the other   Observe his verbal and non-
   says (facts and feelings)   verbal behaviour
7. Choose a listener response   Give some small and medium
                                   listener responses
8. Choose a new question   Ask a specific factual question
9. Choose a new listener   Some more small and medium
   response   listener responses
10. Choose a new question   Ask a general or specific
                              personal question
11. Choose a new listener   Give a full response this time
    response   (reflection)
12. Choose a listener comment   Share your similar feeling or
                                  experience
13. Choose style of parting   Pay respects, take leave

SUMMARY

In this section we have dealt with listener *comments* both verbal
and non-verbal, such as agreeing and disagreeing, showing
puzzlement and surprise. We have also practised expressing
feelings of similarity and difference, and different kinds of questions we can ask.

HOMEWORK ASSIGNMENT 5

Preparation
Write out a 'Cue Card 5, QUESTIONS', listing the four kinds of
topic (not the examples). Also, during the week, write down some
answers to these questions about yourself, drawing on your diary
of daily activities. They will be used next session. Write out the
task and call this 'Task Card 5, COMMENTS AND QUESTIONS'.

The task

1. Carry out the conversation, observation and listening tasks (Cards 1 to 4).
2. While the other person talks, use some of the following listener comments, verbally and non-verbally:

    Agree/disagree
    Pleased/displeased
    Interested/bored
    Puzzled
    Surprised

3. When the other is silent, ask open-ended questions from the topic list:

    (a) ask a *general* (G) question
    (b) ask a *specific* (S) question
    (c) ask a *feeling* (F) belief or opinion-seeking question

Speaking

To hold a conversation, we need to do some listening and some speaking. We have dealt with some of the listening skills, now we move on to speaking skills.

TALKING ABOUT THINGS IN GENERAL

We all have experience and knowledge of all sorts of things. We draw on this kind of information when we talk to each other. However, some people think that what they know just isn't important enough to talk about, so they keep quiet. In fact most ordinary conversations are about fairly unimportant, everyday things, like what happened at work this afternoon, or about a film on the telly, or about the bus being late yet again. This is because 'having a chat' isn't for exchanging important information but simply for maintaining and enjoying a friendly relationship. Below we give a list of suggested topics for you to talk about (it is the same list as for topics for questions).

Exercise 20

1. Pick a topic (below)
2. Recall a situation (consult your diary)
3. Talk about it

Conversation – topics and examples

Topics	*Examples*
1. Anything you have been involved in today/yesterday/weekend/last week etc.	What I did or what happened to me today/yesterday etc.

2. Things you are, do, or belong to
   (i) home   (ii) work
  (iii) travel   (iv) hobbies,
   (v) social   spare-time interests
	What I do at work, home, socially. What my hobbies are. Where I have travelled.

3. Things you might have in common with the other person
   (i) being 'here'
  (ii) places you know (pub, museums, etc.)
  (iii) things you have seen (films, shows, etc.)
  (iv) general interests (cars, hi-fi)
   (v) people you know
	What I am doing 'here'. Pubs I have been to. Films I have seen, etc.

4. Current topics (local and national)
   (i) news, gossip (housing shortage, bus services, etc.)
  (ii) sport   (iii) personalities
  (iv) forthcoming events
	What has happened locally, e.g. how the local football team is doing. Prices.

TALKING ABOUT THINGS IN DETAIL

In conversation we usually start with a general statement, to introduce the topic, and then move on to the details. For instance, we might start with 'I went away for the weekend' and then go on to describe the journey, place visited and so on. This makes our conversation more interesting.

Exercise 21
1. Pick a topic (or wait for a question)
2. Recall a situation
3. Introduce it in general terms
4. Describe it in detail

TALKING ABOUT OUR FEELINGS AND OPINIONS

In conversation we not only give people information about what we've done and experienced (e.g. 'I went away for the weekend...')

but also what we feel and believe about those things (e.g. 'Had a lovely time').

Exercise 22
1. Pick a topic (or wait for a question)
2. Recall a situation
3. Note your feeling, belief or opinion about it
4. Describe it in general terms
5. Describe it in specific terms
6. Describe your feeling, belief or opinion about it

DISCLOSING FEELINGS NON-VERBALLY

We not only *tell* the listener what we think and believe – we also *show* him, by non-verbal expressions.

Exercise 23
As exercise 22, except
6. Express your feelings about it, and accompany this with facial and vocal expression.

Revision

In this section we have dealt with some of the basic skills of speaking – thinking of topics, introducing them, giving details and expressing our feelings and opinions. This helps us to say more, and to be more interesting to the listener.

Now we can combine the listener and speaker skills in another revision exercise. This takes the form of a conversation between two, one taking the role of *listener*, the other of *speaker*, and then swapping over. The steps are given below.

Exercise 24

A		B
LISTENER Decisions	ACTIONS	SPEAKER Decisions
1. Choose a question →	Ask general question, topic 1.	
	Give general, factual answer, topic 1	← Choose a response

2. Choose another → Ask specific question,
   question   topic 1

                        Give specific factual ← Choose another
                        answer, topic 1   response

3. Choose a listener → Give attention
   response   feedback

                        Give more, specific, ← Continue response
                        factual information,
                        topic 1

4. Choose another → Ask 'feeling' question,
   question   topic 1

                        Give 'feeling'   ← Choose another
                        disclosure   response

5. Choose another → Give reflection
   listener response

                        Disclose more feeling ← Continue response
                        about topic 1

6. Choose another → Give attention feedback
   listener response

7. Choose another → Ask general question,
   question   topic 2 or specific question
                        about another aspect
                        of topic 1

                        Give general factual ← Choose a response
                        answer, topic 2.

After reaching step 7, return to step 2 and repeat the sequence
on the next topic.

HOMEWORK ASSIGNMENT 6

Preparation

Write out a 'Cue Card 6, TOPICS', listing the topics from Exercise
20. Write out the task (below) on another card and call this 'Task
Card 6, SPEAKING.' With the help of the instructor, write out a
CHANGE CARD, and list the elements of your behaviour you'd like
to change.

The task

1. Carry out the previous tasks, Cards 1 to 5 (Conversation (1),
   Observation (2), Listening (2)).

2. When the other asks a question, or is silent, select and talk about a topic

   (a) in general terms
   (b) in detail
   (c) express your opinion or feelings about it

3. Control or correct the behaviours listed on your CHANGE CARD, and tick them off if you are successful.

Meshing

We have practised some of the skills of listeners and some of the skills of speakers. Normally we do a bit of both, but if we don't do this smoothly, the conversation can break down. This section is about keeping a conversation going smoothly – which we call meshing.

FLOW

In conversation people talk about similar things – they will have a topic in common, or an opinion or belief in common. If they don't have something in common to talk about, then the conversation becomes very disjointed and confusing.

Exercise 25

Partner A	Partner B
1. Speak about a topic	Respond with a *similar* topic and feeling
2. Speak about another topic	Respond with similar topic but *different* information or feeling
3. Speak about another topic	Respond with *different* topic but *similar* feeling

TIMING

The next thing in running a conversation smoothly is to get the timing right – so that there aren't a lot of interruptions or long silences.

Exercise 26

A	B
1. Speak about a topic	1. Wait until the other finishes
	2. Choose a response
	3. Respond promptly

TURN-TAKING

Sometimes people find it difficult to get the timing right because they don't know how to hand the conversation over or how to take it up. There are special signals for doing these things.

Exercise 27

A	B
1. Speak about a topic	
2. Hand over the conversation, using non-verbal cues (ii) below	Take up the conversation using (iii) or (v)

Exercise 28

A	B
1. Speak about a topic	
2. Try to hand over the conversation verbally, using (i)	Resist the hand-over using (x) or (xi)

Turn-taking signals

Handing over.   Meaning: 'I've finished; over to you'
   (i)   Ask question and continue looking. Lean forward
   (ii) As you finish talking, look at other person, and then look down or away
         Stop gesturing
         Change voice pitch on last word or two
         Use concluding phrase
         Don't start new phrase

Taking up.   Meaning: 'Please finish; I want to speak'
   (iii)   Prepare other that you are going to speak
   (iv) *or* Withhold any response until other stops speaking, and then take up conversation
   (v) *or* Use simple reflection, picking up a word or phrase, but then keep the floor

(vi) *or* Interrupt and begin strongly, avoid speech errors and just keep talking

(vii) *or* In group, get speaker's attention by body shifts and orientation, then use (iii), (v) or (vi)

(viii) *or* Interrupt other person during a pause for thought

Suppressing a turn-claim.   Meaning: 'I'm carrying on'

(ix)   As you reach a point, don't pause, don't look back at other, continue gesturing, talk louder

Resisting a hand-over.   Meaning: 'You carry on'

(x)   Use a listener response and keep looking at other

(xi) *or* Ask question or turn other's question round, then continue looking at other.

SUMMARY

To make a conversation flow smoothly, we have to have something in common to talk about, we have to get the timing right, and we have to know how to take the conversation up and hand it over.

HOMEWORK ASSIGNMENT 7

Preparation
Write out the list of turn-taking signals and call this 'Cue Card 7, TURN-TAKING'. Write out the task below and call this 'Task Card 7, MESHING'. Change, if necessary, the list on your CHANGE CARD.

The task
1. Carry out the previous tasks, Cards 1 to 6, Conversation (1), Observation (2), Listening (1), Questions (1), Speaking (1).
2. When the other person stops speaking, respond with
   (a) similar topic, similar feeling
   (b) similar feeling, different topic
3. When the other person stops speaking, take up the conversation and respond in good time.
4. When you finish speaking, hand over the conversation.

Expression of attitudes

So far we have dealt with basic conversation – the exchange of information, opinions, feelings and so on, between two or more people. But something else goes on between two people in conversation which is not usually talked about. This is the expression of attitudes – how we feel about each other. There are two main attitudes (or styles): friendliness against unfriendliness, and assertiveness (or dominance) as against submissiveness. In this section we shall learn how to express friendliness and assertiveness while we speak and listen.

CHOOSING A STYLE

While conversing we should observe the other's attitude and choose a style or attitude which is similar to, or different from, the other's depending on how we feel about him. If the other is cold, we can choose to be cold, or we can choose some other style – dominance, warmth, etc.

Exercise 29

A	B
1. Talk about a topic in a → friendly style	1. Notice the style and identify the topic
	↓
	2. Talk about a similar topic
2. Notice the style of response ←	in a similar style
and topic discussed	
↓	
3. Repeat the moves *or* choose a different style (e.g. cold)	

CHOOSING FOR EFFECT

The style of behaviour of one person affects the behaviour of the other. If you are cold, the other is likely to be cold. If you are warm, the other is likely to be warm in response, and so on. In the next exercise, we think about how we want to affect the other.

Exercise 30

A	B
1. Decide how you want to affect the other (e.g. keep him friendly)	_____

2. Choose a style you think
   will have this effect, e.g.　———————
   friendliness, and talk about
   a topic in this way　　　　→ 1. Identify topic and attitude

   　　　　　　　　　　　　　　　2. Decide how he wants to
   　　　　　　　　　　　　　　　　　affect you, e.g. keep you
   　　　　　　　　　　　　　　　　　friendly

   　　　　　　　　　　　　　　　3. Decide how you want to
   　　　　　　　　　　　　　　　　　affect him, e.g. maintain
   　　　　　　　　　　　　　　　　　his friendliness, and talk
   　　　　　　　　　　　　　　　　　about the same topic in
3. Identify other's topic and　←　this style
   attitude and repeat the moves.

Exercise 31　Revision
As exercise 30, with the following alternative styles:

A	B
Coldness	1. Warmth *or*
	2. Assertiveness and warmth
Assertiveness	Assertiveness
Submissiveness	Warmth

Social routines

So far, we have dealt with basic conversation skills. But in daily
life we face many more problems. For instance, what is the best
way to start a conversation with a stranger – or to end one when
we want to? What is the best way to make a difficult request, such
as a date, or a favour? How do we handle someone who thinks we
have wronged them in some way? How do we assert ourselves
when someone has wronged us? How can we best show our
appreciation or affection for someone? And so on. In this section
we deal with the appropriate 'social routines' – or how-to-do-it
steps – that are conventional and accepted in our society, for
handling such situations.

GREETINGS

Greetings are so important that conversations would hardly
be possible without them. Failure to use them means that we won't

be able to start conversations; we will insult the other if we fail
to respond to his greeting, and he will not be inclined to greet us
again.

Exercise 32   Interaction greeting

Supplied situation:	A and B have met once before and now find themselves face to face at a party and want to get to know each other
Goal:	Start a conversation
Action:	1. Greet at a distance by brief eye contact and one or more of the following: eyebrow 'flash', brief smile, wave, head nod, brief verbal greeting
	2. If greeting returned: look away while approaching other, then look up; take up a position facing the other person, smile, present hand and follow this by longer, verbal greeting (including use of other's name), handshake, conventional question or statement of respects
	3. Start conversation with a 'bridging' phrase and 'GSF' questions routine, while settling into an appropriate position and orientation
Problem situation:	

Exercise 33   Passing greeting

Supplied situation:	A and B are nodding acquaintances and are passing each other
Goal:	Show mutual respect without getting involved in conversation
Action:	Brief mutual glance, plus one or more of the following: eyebrow 'flash', brief smile, wave, headnod, brief verbal greeting
Problem situation:	

Exercise 34 'Non-greeting'

Supplied situation:	A and B are complete strangers passing in the street
Goal	Show respect and mutual trust without social contact
Action:	Brief mutual looking, then look away. No other change in activity
Problem situation:	

PARTINGS

Partings are equally important. Failure to use them can lead to: the other feeling insulted or rejected; failure to end an unwanted conversation and being 'trapped'.

Exercise 35

Supplied situation:	A and B in the previous sketch have conversed for a few minutes and wish to part in order to talk to other guests
Goal:	End conversation decisively but without awkwardness
Action:	1. Start separation (break gaze, begin positioning for departure, turn away, make verbal comment justifying departure)
	2. If separation accepted, bid farewell (major departure movements, eye contact, smile, handshake, verbal respects)
	3. Part from other (move away, farewell gesture, verbal parting, break gaze, end gesture)
Problem situation:	

REQUESTS

Most people feel inhibited about asking certain things of others, like borrowing something, asking a favour or a date, for fear of giving offence or being turned down. This causes some to hold back and feel frustrated and ineffective. Others make their requests wrongly, and *do* cause the reactions they dread. Here is one accepted way of making a request.

Exercise 36

Supplied situation:	A's car is broken down and he has an important appointment to keep. He goes up to his friend B
Goal:	To borrow B's car without causing embarrassment or insult
Action:	1. Use non-verbal 'immediacy' cues, explain situation, make request direct and to the point
	2a. If other complies, offer appreciation verbally and non-verbally
	2b. If other refuses with apology, minimise request and offer appreciation: 'Never mind, thanks anyway.'
Problem situation:	

APPROACHING STRANGERS

People also feel anxious about approaching strangers, for fear of saying the wrong thing, appearing silly or forward, and of being rejected. There are conventional and accepted ways of approaching strangers, which if used will nearly always avoid these problems.

Exercise 37   Access in private

Supplied situation:	A is a complete stranger in a new club. He goes up to the bar, where a member is standing
Goal:	To get into conversation with the member
Action:	1. Turn head to face other, make brief eye contact, social smile, brief greeting
	2. If returned, make request for information (e.g. what are the prices like here?)
	3. Make self-introduction as an aside ('By the way I'm . . . ') with justification ('I've just joined')
	4. Exchange information about self – work, home, etc. ('Do you live near here? I live . . .')

Problem situation:

access skills in social clubs
Introductions
'Priming' introductions
Self-introductions
Joining in activity
Setting situation up

Exercise 38   Access in public

Supplied situation:	A goes into pub. He goes up to bar where someone is standing
Goal:	To start a conversation
Action:	1. Make verbal request for information or conventional aside (e.g. 'What nice weather'), turn head, make eye contact, give social smile
	2. If responded to, use follow-up question (e.g. 'Wonder how long it'll last?' or 'This your local?')
	3. Exchange information with other about self

Problem situation:

access skills in pubs, coffee bars, etc.
Requests for and offers of
   information
   advice
   favours
Conventional asides about
   the weather
   whatever is happening at the moment
Follow-up questions or disclosures about
   the topic introduced
   'this' place (conditions, service etc.)
   the people here (noisy, crowded)
   the other's connection with this place

OFFERING PRAISE, HELP AND OTHER KINDS OF SUPPORT

Often people want to offer praise and help to someone they like, but do not do so because they think it out of place or feel that they are not important enough to make such gestures, or simply do not know how to do it. There are also accepted and conventional ways of offering praise and help, which virtually always bring pleasure to the other and which are in any case often expected. Failure to make offers of this kind may leave the other feeling hurt.

Exercise 39   Congratulating

Supplied situation:	A goes up to his friend B, who has announced his engagement
Goal:	To congratulate B
Action:	1. Congratulate B (non-verbal 'immediacy' cues including handshake, happy expression, verbal 'congratulations' and reason for this) 2. Follow-up question about the engagement – when date of wedding, etc.
Problem situation:	

Exercise 40   Offering help

Supplied situation:	B has an appointment to keep and his car has broken down; A has a car
Goal:	To offer help
Action:	1. Make the offer and give reasons for offering 2. Confirm offer, possibly insisting if appropriate 3. Minimise the 'sacrifice', emphasise pleasure of doing a favour
Problem situation:	

'MAKING GOOD' (REMEDIAL ROUTINES)

When we take some initiative, there is always the risk we will upset someone who thinks we have done them wrong, or get rejected or rebuffed, often unfairly or inadvertently. We often don't make it up with the other, perhaps because we are afraid to or don't know how to do it. Again, there are well-accepted ways of 'making good', which can go a long way to restore the situation.

Exercise 41   Explaining

Supplied situation :   B blames A for not helping him out of a
                       difficult situation, but A is innocent – he
                       did not get the message
Goal :   To deny all blame
Action :   Use non-verbal assertion cues, verbal
                       account of true situation and explanation
                       of innocence
Problem situation :

Exercise 42   Apologising

Supplied situation :   B rightly blames A for upsetting B's
                       mother
Goal :   Remedy the insult without losing face.
Action :   1. Non-verbal 'immediacy' cues, serious
                          expression, verbal apology, acknowl-
                          edgement of fault, account minimising
                          blame, expression of chagrin
                       2. If other demands further apology,
                          repeat apology briefly and change
                          subject
                       3. If other still demands further apology
                          use assertive cues, refuse further
                          apology, terminate interaction or
                          change subject
Problem situation :

Exercise 43   Saving face

Supplied situation :   A wants to ask B for a date
Goal :   Ask for a date but be prepared to handle
                       a rebuff without embarrassment
Action :   1. Greet B
                       2. Hold conversation
                       3. Make request for date directly, with
                          use of non-verbal 'immediacy' cues
                       4. If other gives excuse, offer different
                          date
                       5. If other gives excuse, accept excuse at
                          face value, repeat invitation but leave
                          date open ('I'll ring you'). Maintain
                          positive attitude

ASSERTION

Many people are not very good at asserting themselves when someone has done them wrong, for instance by jumping ahead in a queue, interrupting in conversation, failing to fulfil a service one has paid for, making unreasonable demands, and so on. Failure to assert oneself in such situations does damage to one's self-respect and quite often to one's pocket too. People often fail to assert themselves because they are afraid of the consequences, perhaps they have previously done it in the wrong way. There are effective ways of asserting oneself which usually overcome these problems.

Exercise 44   Assertion

Supplied situation:	B rudely pushes in front of A and calls for service
Goal:	To restore the situation and get an apology
Action:	1. Check out possible explanation and excuses
	2. Make implicit request by non-verbal assertive cues, statement of the facts, rhetorical question, etc.
	3. If unsuccessful, make explicit request
	4. If unsuccessful, make explicit demand and possible threat
Problem situation:	

Exercise 45   Refusal

Supplied situation:	B persists in asking A for a date, who is against the idea
Goal:	To refuse in the face of persistence
Action:	1. Check the reasonableness of the request
	2. Imply refusal by non-verbal means (no 'immediacy' cues) and use of excuse
	3. Repeat 2 if unsuccessful
	4. Make refusal more explicit by withholding excuse

5. Make refusal explicit, point out he is 'pushing his luck' and threaten reprisals (if appropriate)

Problem situation:

Exercise 46   Revision
1. Describe a problem situation
2. Practise the skilled response suggested

Tactics

Many of the skills practised in earlier sessions are difficult to use in real-life social encounters, because we invariably fall back on life-long bad habits, perhaps backing down or opting out, when the going gets tough. So one problem is: We may know what to do, but by the time we remember to do it, it is too late. There are ways of breaking down old bad habits, and making conscious choices at the right moments. There are three points to remember: Think of alternatives, choose the best one, use it at the right moment.

Exercise 47   Alternatives
1. Consider the problem situation supplied by the therapist
2. Suggest as many alternative responses as you can think of
3. Evaluate each of these as right, wrong or neutral
   Evaluate others suggested to you
4. Choose one of the best responses and practise this
5. Give a problem situation of your own and work through these steps again

Exercise 48   More alternatives
1. Start a conversation with your partner
2. Stop upon request and think of as many alternative responses as you can
3. Select one of the better of these and continue

alternative conversation responses
At each choice point in a conversation a number of alternative responses are possible. Here is one example:

Alternative responses to a non-verbal hand-over

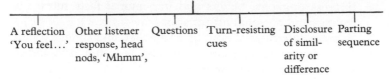

A reflection 'You feel...'	Other listener response, head nods, 'Mhmm',	Questions	Turn-resisting cues	Disclosure of similarity or difference	Parting sequence

Strategies

In addition to the decisions we make about tactics within a conversation, we also have to decide on a plan or strategy for a whole conversation or series of conversations. What we decide upon depends on what we want in the situation, and on our repertoire of skills.

REWARDING OTHERS

One goal may be to get the other interested, talking and responding more, to feel more friendly towards you.

Exercise 49   Rewarding strategy
1. Pick someone out and get relevant information if possible
2. On sighting, greet him
3. Ask a few questions (GSF question routine)
4. Give full listener responses
5. Give personal information and express feelings of similarity
6. Be expressive (non-verbal signals)
7. Mesh smoothly
8. Offer praise and help
9. Use 'making good' routines if necessary

CONTROLLING OTHERS

Another goal may be to get the other to talk less, or about different things, and reduce his control of you and the situation.

Exercise 50 Controlling strategy
1. Select 'target' person, get relevant information, if possible
2. On sighting, greet him
3. Ask many questions
4. Use fewer listener responses

5. Speak at length
6. Express opinions, beliefs and impersonal facts more than feelings and personal information
7. Express *differences* of opinion and belief, and change topics
8. Use non-verbal emotion expression less, but non-verbal speech accompaniments more
9. Use dominance cues (especially vocal and postural)
10. Use interruptions and non-response, hand-over and take-up cues, but suppress turn offers and resist turn claims
11. Make requests, give advice, refusals, assert rights, resist apologies
12. Use negative attitude cues if appropriate

PRESENTING SELF

Another goal may be to make a good impression on the other about the sort of person you are.

Exercise 51   Presenting self
1. Prepare physical appearance
2. Maintain eye contact, high muscular tonus, face-to-face orientation, voice volume and clarity
3. Mask verbal and non-verbal expression of negative emotional states with positive and socially sanctioned expressions
4. Make verbal disclosures suggestive of status, and withhold negative information
5. Be rewarding
6. Be controlling

COMBINING TACTICS AND STRATEGIES

In this last exercise we want you to practise strategies and tactics together. This is a complicated exercise, so the instructors may divide you into pairs and give you a script to act out as a first step. Then you will be asked to think up a situation for yourselves.

Exercise 52

A	B
1. Adopt an attitude to B (e.g. superior)	————————
2. Decide on an appropriate behavioural strategy to express this (e.g. controlling)	————————
3. At this point use a tactic → that fits into your overall strategy (i.e. to control)	Observe A's tactics. What strategy do you think he is using
4. ————————————	Decide on your own strategy (e.g. counter-control)
5. Observe B's tactics. What ← strategy is he using?	At this point respond with a tactic that fits into your chosen strategy

Repeat Steps 2 to 5

HOMEWORK ASSIGNMENTS

The instructors will set homework assignments where they have not already been prepared in this handbook.

Author index

Subject index

Contemporary Community Health Series

LONG-TERM CHILDHOOD ILLNESS
Harry A. Sultz, Edward R. Schlesinger, William E. Mosher, and Joseph
G. Feldman

MARRIAGE AND MENTAL HANDICAP: *A Study of Subnormality
in Marriage*
Janet Mattinson

A METHOD OF HOSPITAL UTILIZATION REVIEW
Sidney Shindell and Morris London

METHODOLOGY IN EVALUATING THE QUALITY OF
MEDICAL CARE: *An Annotated Selected Bibliography, 1955–1968*
Isidore Altman, Alice J. Anderson, and Kathleen Barker
Out of print

MIGRANTS AND MALARIA IN AFRICA
R. Mansell Prothero
Out of print

THE PSYCHIATRIC HALFWAY HOUSE: *A Handbook of Theory
and Practice*
Richard D. Budson

A PSYCHIATRIC RECORD MANUAL FOR THE HOSPITAL
Dorothy Smith Keller

RACISM AND MENTAL HEALTH
Charles V. Willie, Bernard M. Kramer, and Bertram S. Brown, Editors

SOCIAL SKILLS AND MENTAL HEALTH
Peter Trower, Bridget Bryant, and Michael Argyle

THE SOCIOLOGY OF PHYSICAL DISABILITY AND
REHABILITATION
Gary L. Albrecht, Editor

THE STYLE AND MANAGEMENT OF A PEDIATRIC
PRACTICE
Lee W. Bass, and Jerome H. Wolfson

M